Stopping the Insanity

Albert Einstein once said that the definition of insanity is "doing the same thing over and over again and expecting different results." Boy, if this is true, I went nuts a long time ago! But somewhere along the way I came to my senses by realizing I had to make a choice: keep living the same way I'd been living and spend the rest of my life on a roller-coaster ride I'd never get off or get real and make some drastic changes in lifestyle that would prolong my life, if not save it altogether.

My weight will continue to be a lifelong battle, but at least I'm prepared to face it head-on and slay the dragon. I know it'll take hard work, discipline, perseverance, and persistence. If I had a choice between going on a twelve-mile run or sitting at home in front of the fire reading a book, I would prefer the book, but that isn't going to keep me in shape. So when I weigh the options there's one thing I know for sure—I no longer identify myself as the fat, jolly weatherman. And I'm never goin' back.

NEVER GOIN' BACK

Winning the Weight-loss Battle for Good

Al Roker

with Laura Morton

 NEW AMERICAN LIBRARY

NEW AMERICAN LIBRARY
Published by the Penguin Group
Penguin Group (USA) LLC, 375 Hudson Street,
New York, New York 10014

USA | Canada | UK | Ireland | Australia | New Zealand | India | South Africa | China
penguin.com
A Penguin Random House Company

Published by New American Library, a division of Penguin Group (USA) LLC. Previously published in a
New American Library hardcover edition.

First New American Library Trade Paperback Printing, January 2014

REGISTERED TRADEMARK—MARCA REGISTRADA

NEW AMERICAN LIBRARY TRADE PAPERBACK ISBN: 978-0-451-41494-6

THE LIBRARY OF CONGRESS HAS CATALOGUED THE HARDCOVER EDITION OF THIS TITLE AS FOLLOWS:
Roker, Al, 1954–
Never goin' back: winning the weight-loss battle for good/Al Roker with Laura Morton.
p.   cm.
ISBN 978-0-451-41493-9
1. Roker, Al, 1954– —Health.   2. Weight loss.   3. Reducing diets.
4. Compulsive eating.   I. Morton, Laura, 1964–   II. Title.   III. Title: Never goin' back.
RM222.2.R6273 2013
613.2'5—dc23   2012031429

Printed in the United States of America
10 9 8 7 6 5 4 3 2 1

Set in Chaparall Pro
Designed by Sabrina Bowers

PUBLISHER'S NOTE
While the author has made every effort to provide accurate telephone numbers, Internet addresses and other contact information at the time of publication, neither the publisher nor the author assumes any responsibility for errors, or for changes that occur after publication. Further, publisher does not have any control over and does not assume any responsibility for author or third-party Web sites or their content.

The recipes contained in this book are to be followed exactly as written. The publisher is not responsible for your specific health or allergy needs that may require medical supervision. The publisher is not responsible for any adverse reactions to the recipes contained in this book.

I'd like to dedicate this book to my dad, Al Roker Sr. Without your inspiration, Dad, I would never have taken the steps to get on this path that I'm on. I also dedicate it to my children, Courtney, Leila and Nicky. You guys are the reasons Pop-Pop wanted me to get healthy. And finally, to my wife, Deborah. Your love and support continue to give me the freedom and the courage to continue this journey. I love you all.

AL ROKER JR.

Contents

NEVER GOIN' BACK

Introduction

July 2001

My father had been at Memorial Sloan-Kettering hospital in New York City for about a week, battling his final stages of lung cancer. Although he had been a smoker early in his life, he had given up cigarettes cold turkey some thirty-five years prior to his cancer diagnosis. So when he was told that he had stage four lung cancer, I wasn't emotionally prepared. Our entire family was shaken up and took his diagnosis very hard.

Al Roker Sr. was the rock of our family. Even though he was a talented artist, in the mid-1950s, it was difficult for a young African-American male to get a job in the commercial art industry. After a short stint at a low-paying apprentice job with no chance for advancement, with a young wife and a new baby to feed, Dad got a job driving a New York City bus.

He would do that for almost twenty years, always looking for the next step up. Eventually he made dispatcher, then chief dispatcher, and then he was promoted up and into management with the Metropolitan Transit Authority, reaching the rank of Inspector.

We were all so proud of him. His drive and determination rubbed off on his children. We would strive to make him and our mother as proud of us as we were of them.

When he retired, he was excited and determined to enjoy life. My dad found pleasure in being with his wife and his grandchildren, and in his lifelong hobby of deep-sea fishing. He cultivated a newfound love of jazz, started a mentoring program for middle schoolers at a local public school and walked with a group of fellow retirees at the local mall.

But all of that was now behind him. His entire future had now collapsed into being measured by weeks, if not days.

Every day I made it a point to stop in, first thing in the morning, before heading to the studio to do the *Today* show. We'd visit, and then about six twenty a.m., I'd head on to Studio 1-A in Rockefeller Plaza, where the show goes live at seven a.m. On my way home in the afternoon, I'd head straight back to the hospital to spend more time with him—*time,* something I had all but taken for granted until my father got sick.

Time.

Why hadn't I gone fishing with him more than a handful of times, and why didn't I come by the house more often? I always thought I would have plenty of *time*.

My father was always healthy as a horse. Mom was the one who had beaten lung cancer and breast cancer and survived two heart valve replacements! Dad almost never got sick. Now he was dying and I had just about run out of time with the man I cherished most in life.

There was nowhere near enough time.

"Son," my dad said one day, "I'd do anything for more time. I wanted to make fifty years of marriage with your mom so, yeah, I'm pissed about that."

It was kind of funny, actually. My father always liked things well-ordered and tidy. He was sixty-nine years old and had been married forty-nine years. To him, seventy and fifty felt neater—more complete.

I knew my dad was going to die. There was no hope that he could possibly recover. I did my best to hold myself together until one morning I simply couldn't hide my grief about losing him. I started crying, and being the incredible father he was, he comforted me.

He said he was proud of the life he had lived—that he'd had a good run. He told me he was proud of his children and he loved his grandchildren more than life itself. Hearing my father speak that way was simply more than I could bear; it was all so final. My tears kept coming. I could tell that my father had something important he wanted to say.

"Look, we both know that I'm not going to be here to help you raise my grandkids, so that means it is up to you to make sure *you* will be there for your kids."

I could feel my heart begin beating faster with every word he uttered because I knew what he was driving at. My father and I had been around the horn too many times to count on the subject of my weight and overall health. For whatever reason, no matter how many times I said I'd lose the weight, I couldn't—or wouldn't, or did only to gain it back again.

"Promise me that you are going to lose the weight."

I tried to play it off like it was no big deal. "Who, me? I'm fine! Don't worry about me, Dad."

• •

3

I could tell he was really struggling to get the words out now. "No, not good enough. I want you to swear to God that you're going to lose the weight."

I realized there was really only one respectable thing to do—promise him I would lose the weight.

Ugh.

Now, I don't know if you've ever had to make a deathbed promise to someone you love, but if you have, you know the kind of guilt and massive responsibility I felt in that moment. And if you haven't, let me assure you, it was heavy—heavier than me, and I was damn big. I couldn't say a word. It wasn't that I didn't want to, because I did, but I was hesitant. Nothing I could say would mean all that; I had said it all before, without ever doing the work to permanently change my mind-set and lose the weight for good.

So, I promised him I would lose the weight. Still, that wasn't good enough for him. He wanted me to swear to God that I was going to lose the weight—and so I did.

"Dad, I swear to God I am going to lose this weight."

"I am going to hold you to that, son. You don't want to make me angry."

Trust me, I *didn't* want to get him angry.

I remember when I was twelve years old and my folks had gotten me a brand-new Sting-Ray bicycle for my birthday. It had a banana seat and a metallic blue paint job. I loved that bike!

Well, one Saturday afternoon, some young thugs from outside our neighborhood came cruising through. They surrounded me, punched me a few times, knocked me off the bike and took it. My pride was hurt more than anything else, but when I got home and told my dad what happened, I saw a look come over him that I had never seen. "Get in the car. Let's go look for your bike," he said through clenched teeth. He got behind the wheel and I got in on the passenger's side and we went looking for these guys and my bike.

After around fifteen minutes of driving around, I noticed a dishtowel wrapped around something sitting on the seat between the two of us. I unwrapped an edge of the towel and saw a steak knife! Dad was going to *find that bike* and was prepared to fight anyone who got in his way. That's who my dad was. We never actually found the bike but I discovered I loved my father that day even more than I knew because of his willingness to protect who and what he loved.

He was also the same man who cried when he deposited his firstborn son at the dorm on my first day of college. Everything he was made me who I am.

And now that was all about to go away.

So on the morning I made that promise to my dad, I left the hospital thinking about what he had said—a lot. I don't usually get distracted when I am on the air, but his words echoed in my mind the entire show. I was so upset about my promise to lose weight, in fact, that I had two grilled cheese and bacon sandwiches for lunch. My mantra at the time was "When in doubt, eat."

When I returned to the hospital that afternoon, Dad was out of his bed, sitting up in a chair.

"Hey, old man, how you doing?" I said, but there was no response. He was just looking off into space. One of the nurses came in and told me he'd suddenly stopped talking earlier that day.

"Why?" I asked. The nurse said she would get one of his doctors to explain what was going on. You know it's always bad news when someone says they want to get someone else to explain things to you. In other words: "Here comes bad news and they don't pay me enough to put up with the grief you will probably give me!"

When the doctor arrived, he said that my dad's cancer had spread to his brain. It was affecting his ability to speak and would likely impair his motor functions very soon.

As I helped the doctor and the nurse transfer my father back into bed, he lost control of his bowels. He couldn't say anything, but the look on his face was heartbreaking. My father, the strongest man I knew, both physically and emotionally, was leaving. And there was nothing I could do about it.

A couple of weeks earlier, planning for this moment, my family had made the decision to move Dad, when the time came, to Calvary Hospital in the Bronx. It is the world leader in palliative care, run by the Archdiocese of New York.

Two days later we transferred him to Calvary, where angels do heaven's work on earth and where he would spend his final days. My brother and sisters all came to say good-bye to their father. Our spouses sat by his bed. His grandchildren were there. And we all hugged and held my mother as she watched her husband slip away.

That week was a blur, but I can tell you just about the entire menu at the Calvary cafeteria. I was aware that I was using food to ease the pain, but I didn't care. As we all kept vigil by my dad's side, I kept thinking about the promise I had made to him and wondering, "How the hell am I going to do this?"

CHAPTER ONE

A Portly Kid from Queens

I was born in Queens, New York, in 1954. I am the oldest of six kids, three boys and three girls. Three of us are the biological children of my parents and three were adopted through foster care. I am one of the biological kids, along with a sister who's six years younger and a "baby" brother, who is seventeen years younger than me. Although I was a premature baby, weighing in at four pounds, ten ounces, at a certain point very early in my life, I just started eating and never stopped. I suppose my family heritage added to my genetic lot in life. Both of my parents came from families who loved to eat. My mom, Isabel, also known as "Izzy," was half-Jamaican, and my dad was from the Bahamas. Dad looked like a young Sidney Poitier, who happened to be from Exuma, the same island in the Bahamas where my father's family was from. When my dad was younger, people often did a double take when they saw him driving his white Plymouth Valiant station wagon—the same car Sidney Poitier drove in *Lilies of the Field*.

My parents met at John Adams High School in Queens. My mother was one of the first African-American cheerleaders at the school—at the time, a very big deal. She must have loved being a cheerleader because I grew up hearing a constant chant of "Rickity, rackity, shanty town. Who can knock John Adams down? Nobody. Nobody. Absolutely nobody! Yeah, team!" Honestly, I can't believe I still remember her saying that, but I do!

My dad was an affable guy and a really sharp dresser. He was a very good storyteller who enjoyed sharing tales from his younger days. Turns out, my dad was a stone-cold thug! He had friends with names like Deadeye and Jelly Roll. He had a walking stick that had a knife in it.

Yeah, growing up, he was a tough guy. But by the time his children came along, he was a short teddy bear. (I like to say I come from folks built low to the ground, with one leg shorter than the other, the better to lean into the wind and survive hurricanes.) Of my parents, Dad was definitely the gentler one. If you fell and skinned a knee, you went right to Dad. He'd comfort you and give you a big bear hug, whereas Mom was more likely to tell us to stop crying. Her approach was the early version of "man up."

You might say Izzy was the *original* Tiger Mom. She was tough as nails and, unlike a lot of women of her generation, she enjoyed confrontation. To her, it was sport. I knew I was loved by her, but she knew exactly how to needle me, and what drove me crazy.

Whenever she'd come to my house for dinner, just as I was serving the meal, she'd ask, "Is this any good?"

"No, I just spent an hour making you something that tastes like crap!" I'd respond.

Mom loved to banter and was a real joker. She was also honest to a fault and didn't believe in coddling. She taught my younger daughter, Leila, to play checkers as a kid. Most grandparents let the kids win—but not my mom. No way. To her, losing is how you learn. And now I call Leila "little Izzy" because she is so much like my mom. I once overheard her playing Monopoly with some of her friends. She wiped the board. Then one of her friends asked, "Where'd you learn how to play Monopoly?"

"My nana," Leila said with great pride. I couldn't help but smile.

I was what you might call a late bloomer. As hard as this might be to believe today, I didn't talk until I was three and a half years old. Of course, as a family friend pointed out later, I could never get a word in edgewise anyway! My mom did all the talking for me. She was like my PR agent.

Although I was born premature, I think my lack of development was a combination of being extremely shy—something I never really outgrew—and what today might be labeled as a learning disorder. The only thing I had no problems learning was eating. Well, maybe I had one issue I didn't learn, and that was when to stop.

Although my siblings and I have the same father, he was really two different guys over the years. *My* dad drove a bus and was a blue-collar worker. He hustled every day to provide for his family. When I was a young boy, he and a couple of buddies from NYC Transit, as it was then known, opened up a luncheonette in the depot. They made and sold sandwiches in addition to working their regular shifts. My dad was the kind of man who did whatever it took to make sure his family had everything we needed. In a Caribbean family, if you only had two jobs, you were obviously slacking off.

But the drivers *all* had their rackets going to supplement their incomes. For example, there was always someone selling hot merchandise—you know, things they claimed fell off the back of a truck somewhere. In fact, my dad bought my first movie camera, which sparked my initial interest in animation and television, from one of the guys at the depot.

Unlike a lot of men from that era, my father was very demonstrative; he was a big hugger and kisser. When I saw my uncles and cousins, my impulse was to greet them with a bear hug and a kiss, while they usually held out their hands waiting for a handshake. There was a lot of PDA in my parents' household. And I remember coming home from college to find my mother in the kitchen doing dishes.

"How would you feel about another brother or sister?" she asked.

"Are you going to adopt again?"

"No."

"Oh, then we're taking in another foster kid?"

"No . . ." she replied, and then paused.

Not adopting. No foster kid. . . . Oh for the love of . . . I didn't want to think about *that*! They're my parents, for Pete's sake!

Mom always wanted a big family. She was the second youngest of nine kids, so a big family is all she knew. After she had me and my sister, she had trouble getting pregnant, so she and my dad decided to adopt and open their home to numerous foster children over the years. While sometimes people refer to foster or adopted children as half brothers and half sisters, to me they are my siblings. Needless to say, it came as something of a surprise when she got pregnant seventeen years after having me.

By the time my baby brother was born, Dad had transitioned from blue-collar worker to white-collar executive. He had been promoted and was working in management for the New York Transit Authority. He had an office and a secretary and wore a suit to work every day. I always maintain that I had the more fun dad because I got to do more than my kid brother. When my brother went to work with "executive" dad, he got to play with the Xerox machines. When I went to work with "bus driver" dad, I got to play with change machines, pretend to steer the bus and hang with the guys in the depot. Those were some of my favorite days as a kid.

We'd start the day off by going to Goody's for breakfast. Goody's was a luncheonette near where we lived in Rockaway. He always ordered a bacon and egg sandwich on a hard roll. Wanting to be just like him, I'd do the same. We took our breakfast with us and ate it on the way to the depot.

The NYC Transit Authority Fifth Avenue Depot was a combination of train yard and bus garage. To a seven-year-old boy, it was a magical combination. At the start of his shift, Dad would take me into the locker room where he'd change into his uniform. When other bus drivers opened their lockers, GREAT LAND OF PLENTY . . . *Playboy* pinups!! Don't change into that uniform too quickly, Pop.

After boarding his bus, we'd stop at the corner deli. He'd buy me a stack of comic books and a bag of candy to keep me occupied.

I loved playing with the change machines on the buses— remember, this was at a time, looong before MetroCards, when drivers actually made change for passengers. I'd ride on the bus with him for the entire eight-hour shift all along Flatbush Avenue in Brooklyn. I'd see the same people going to work and then coming home at the end of the day. Somewhere around noon, we took our lunch break, and ate whatever my mom packed for us in the two brown paper bags she sent us out the door with early that morning. When we went back to the depot at the end of his shift, there was always a driver tossing a quarter my way so I could buy a candy bar from the vending machine or get an ice cream. "Hey, little Al, here ya go! Go buy something to eat!" Sometimes I'd just get a Yoo-hoo chocolate milk and throw it back at the end of the day like a tall, cold beer.

Because there were six kids, the vibe in my parents' home was mostly controlled chaos. I have no idea how my mother handled six kids without any help. I have three kids and lots of help and sometimes my wife and I *still* have a hard time doing it all! Whenever I asked Mom what her secret was, she always said, "You kids took care of yourselves." I suppose fear was our great motivator because I, for one, never wanted to be on the receiving end of Dad's spankings. It was a different era, but I knew I'd get my butt whupped good if I got out of line or didn't do what I was told. Back then, if someone in the neighborhood saw me do something—anything I shouldn't be doing—they'd discipline me first and then tell my parents. Oh yeah, it takes a village, and back in the Rockaway projects of Queens, New York, our fifth-floor apartment was in the heart of that village.

As our family grew, my parents needed more space than our old two-bedroom apartment, so when I was eleven, they bought a three-bedroom house in a new development we found during one of our weekend family drives to Elmont, Long Island, to visit Gouz Dairy Farm. (Their slogan? GOUZ RHYMES WITH COWS.

• •

Okay, it wasn't *Mad Men*, but hey, I've remembered it all these years!) We loved going to Gouz. There's nothing like the taste of fresh milk straight from the farm. But the best part was their petting zoo. All the parents would drop their kids off to look at the cows, rabbits and chickens while they went to get fresh milk from the dairy counter. And did I mention the limitless free samples of full-fat chocolate milk? Gouz was a magical place for a growing boy with a growing waistline.

Anyway, we'd usually take the Belt Parkway to get to Long Island, but one day the parkway was so backed up that my dad got off to take a shortcut. That's when he spotted the development of semiattached homes. We stopped to look at the model home and it was love at first sight. My folks scraped together two hundred dollars for a down payment on the spot, and six months later, we all moved in. Even though both of my parents are gone, I still own that house. Whenever my kids go back to look at the house, they can't believe that eight of us fit into three rooms and a single bath! I always joke with my kids and tell them that in order to use the bathroom, we had to take a number like we were at a deli counter waiting to place an order.

Although my parents had a lot of mouths to feed, I never went hungry; I just didn't go back for second or third helpings very often. We always made sure that everyone had a fair portion of whatever Mom made to eat. Mom's cooking was hearty— another word for "heavy"—so it was filling *and* fattening. She was a good cook . . . though breakfast really wasn't her strong suit—you know, the oatmeal was always a little too thick and her pancakes were never "light and fluffy." We ate a lot of cereal! Unfortunately, my dad wouldn't buy the brands of cereals I really wanted as a boy, which was pretty much anything with loads of sugar—Sugar Pops, Frosted Flakes and Sugar Smacks. At least the cereal makers were up-front about their products back then—they may as well have put "Yup, you are pouring sugar" on every box!

My dad's philosophy was one box of corn flakes fits all.

You want Frosted Flakes?

Pour some sugar on those Kellogg's Corn Flakes and voilà! You've got your own frosted cereal.

Oh yeah? Well, this cereal box doesn't have a tiger on it. Just some freaky-looking rooster. Where's Tony the Tiger? I loved Tony the Tiger. I thought he was so cool, especially when I watched my morning cartoons and saw him riding in a car with Huckleberry Hound. It didn't get any cooler than that. Neither Sugar Bear nor Snap, Crackle and Pop had a thing on Tony the Tiger! He was. . . . GRRRRREAT!!!!!

When it came to lunch and dinner, Mom never made anything fancy, but her food was always good. She made a great Velveeta and tomato grilled cheese with Campbell's tomato soup. I don't know anyone who *didn't* grow up eating that grilled cheese and tomato soup combination, but something about my mom's version was special—at least to me.

Lunch also brought the first convergence of food and my eventual career, via Soupy Sales, a comedian I grew up watching on TV. He had a kids' show on at noon on ABC. There was a segment called "What's for Lunch?"

"Mom, Soupy is having a tuna patty melt . . ." I'd shout across the kitchen so my mom would make me one, too. Since this was before I started kindergarten, I had a standing lunch date every day with Soupy. I'd eat my lunch glued to his show, wondering what it would be like to be just like him someday.

I gained an early interest in cooking from both of my parents, but my mom was my true inspiration. Whenever she was cooking, I liked helping her out. I enjoyed the process of gathering the food and ingredients, putting it all together and voilà! Like magic there was a delicious meal on the table. The meals in our house were never fancy but they were always delicious.

Sundays were either a pot roast with potatoes or a roasted chicken with green beans. On occasion, Mom might make pork chops or oxtail stew with dumplings. As I've gotten older, I've thought about those meals many times over the years, trying to recall the tastes and flavors I enjoyed so much as a kid. I really loved my mother's cooking. To this day I still crave her macaroni and cheese, her Jamaican black-eyed peas and rice and her amazing corn bread.

It was an unwritten rule in our house to never bother her while she was cooking. The only exception was when she was making her Sweet Potato Poon for the holidays. This was a crustless pie—well, more like a soufflé than a traditional pie—with marshmallows all over the top, which she would finish by putting in the oven to brown. Every year, one of us kids would do something to distract her from opening the oven door so that the marshmallows would catch fire. Then she would yell at us to get out as the smoke detector blared overhead. It wasn't Thanksgiving until that old smoke detector went off.

I am amazed to think she created our huge holiday feasts in our tiny kitchen, using a single oven and a four-burner stove. Thanksgiving brought fourteen or sixteen people into our home. We'd put every leaf in our expandable wooden dining room table, and we'd still need a card table for the extra people who just stopped by.

When it came to food, my mother and I were perfectly simpatico. She used it as a reward and I liked to eat. My rewards ranged from a bag of M&M's to smoked salmon with cream cheese. I didn't have a particularly sophisticated or discriminating palate back then. In fact, one of my favorite snacks was sliced bananas with sour cream, sprinkled with sugar and cinnamon on top.

By the time I was seven or eight years old, I'd gone from being a solid boy to a pretty chubby kid. It seemed as though all of a sudden I was shopping in the husky boys' section of the local department store.

Husky.

Like I was going to be strapped to a dogsled and forced to run the Iditarod.

When I first started gaining weight, I thought it was normal. Lots of other kids in our neighborhood looked just like me, so I didn't have anything else to compare myself to. By the time I was in the seventh grade, I had a real weight problem—but no one ever talked about it. My parents never gave me a hard time or pushed me to get out of the house and do something active. I was one of those kids who liked sitting around reading comic books, tinkering with old TVs or making my own movies. Today, I'd be a video game geek. Thankfully, they didn't have those kinds of devices when I was a kid, so at least I had to focus my creativity on other things.

I went to St. Catherine of Sienna, a Catholic school in St. Albans, Queens. In between seventh grade and eighth grade, I was chosen to take part in a summer program run by the Jesuits for "underprivileged" kids, called the Higher Achievement Program or HAP. Kids who did well in that summer program were offered a full scholarship at a Jesuit high school.

Make no mistake, for a lower-middle-class family, paying for six kids in Catholic school was no joke. But my parents felt it was a better education and worth the sacrifice. Besides offering a great opportunity for a Jesuit education, HAP had a kick-ass free lunch. I was in!

I did well, but because I wasn't the most physically active kid (and did I mention the *really, really* kick-ass free lunch?), I gained a little more weight. Sure, I played some basketball, but lacking height, speed, any dribbling skills, a hook shot or a jumper, I was mostly used to clog the lane.

I was offered a scholarship to Xavier High School in Manhattan. This was a Big Deal. Xavier High School was and is one of the best high schools, public or private, in New York City. It was also, at the time, a military academy, with full military uniforms.

I became painfully aware that I was having a weight issue when I had to get my school uniform and they didn't have any that fit me. The uniforms were very expensive, so graduating students often donated their uniforms to hand down to incoming students like me. But since none of those fit, my parents had to scrape up about three hundred bucks to buy me a new set.

I started high school in the fall of 1968 and I fell right into a routine. When I went to school in Queens, I took a city bus or could walk to school. Now I had to take a bus and a subway into Manhattan, to Sixteenth Street and Sixth Avenue. I would get up around six a.m. and have breakfast, sometimes with my dad, then head into Manhattan to get to school by seven forty-five. Sometimes I would get in early enough to grab a candy bar at the deli down the street from school. For the long trip home I usually had a candy bar or two to fortify me, then a snack during homework and then dinner. Hey, Mom, did the dry cleaner's shrink this uniform? It's feeling a little snug.

As I entered my sophomore year, my parents were concerned I was putting on too much weight. Always a stocky kid, I was moving into the actual heavy category. It was right around this time that my mother received a flyer in the mail from my dad's health insurance company. Like a lot of municipal workers, he belonged to the Health Insurance Plan of Greater New York, or HIP, a precursor to the dreaded health maintenance organization, or HMO. In exchange for free or low-cost health care, you went to clinics. Well, our local HIP office was offering a weight-loss clinic just for teens. Damn you, HIP. You and your outreach to ever-expanding teens.

This "program" was my first organized diet and consisted mainly of celery sticks, cottage cheese and rye crackers. It was basically a rip-off of Weight Watchers. You came in once a week, weighed in and talked about your challenges with a counselor and a group of your peers.

There were two problems.

1. It was very hard to stick with because it was bland and boring and it left me hungry all of the time.

2. The counselor was a woman in her thirties who was overweight herself. I'm going to take advice from her? And then talk to a bunch of kids who all looked like me? This was doomed from the start.

Sure, I lost five pounds initially, but it was so stressful, I began stopping at the candy store by the bus stop on my way home from the meetings and I put the weight right back on.

Now this was just about the time that Bill Cosby introduced his character Fat Albert. As a kid, I was a huge fan of Bill Cosby. The second album I ever bought was his classic *Why Is There Air?* (Just in case you're wondering, the first album I bought was *Al-*

vin and the Chipmunks Sing the Beatles . . . but that's another story!)

Fat Albert first appeared in Cosby's stand-up routine, then in 1969, he showcased the character in a half hour prime-time special entitled *Hey, Hey, Hey, It's Fat Albert*. I remember watching it and being enamored with the animation, before a horrible rush fell over me.

In a split second, I realized that *I was Fat Albert.*

Oh God.

I was black, fat and named . . . gulp . . . Albert!

My life was over.

This was the worst thing that could have happened to me.

My head was spinning from the thought of having to go to school the next day. I panicked, knowing every one of my schoolmates was home watching this special like I was. I tried to come up with a good excuse to avoid going to school the next morning, but none came to mind. My mom would never believe I was suddenly "sick."

The next day, I went into the cafeteria at Xavier, terrified to be there. Of course, not so terrified that I couldn't stop to buy something to eat. Much to my surprise, no one said a word at first. "Well, maybe nobody saw the show," I thought. But within five seconds of that wishful thinking, I heard eight or ten guys shout out, "Hey, hey, hey!"

I could feel my heart hit my toes as I lowered my head in shame.

I spent the rest of that week enduring everyone's imitations of Fat Albert. I did my best to hide my true feelings by laughing along with everyone else, but on the inside, I was dying. I am sure I had been teased before about my weight, but it had never been the subject of a national television show before. This was much worse. I knew I was chunky but I never felt bad about my weight because I wasn't unusual. I had friends in school who were the same size I was, so I didn't give it a lot of thought. It's not like people stopped and pointed at me for being so fat. My focus wasn't really on my weight so much as it was on the things that were of interest to me—especially as I got older.

Xavier High School fed my love of media. I did all kinds of extracurricular activities. Athletics, not so much. But I joined the newspaper staff and the yearbook. I was on the Audio Visual Squad. (If there was a projector that lost its loop, I could rethread it at a moment's notice!) We even had a closed-circuit TV channel that I worked on. To support my burgeoning love of film and photography, which needed a steady supply of cameras and accessories, I knew I needed to augment my allowance, so I got an after-school job.

This was not just any job. For a food-obsessed teenager, this was a dream job. It was literally right across the street from Xavier's back door. It was a place called A to Z Vending. It was a small vending machine company, and it was my job to fill the boxes that the guys would take to the vending machines in offices across Manhattan.

Can you comprehend the magnitude of this job? Every day I went up and down the many long aisles that were lined with every conceivable snack and candy bar known to man in 1969. Vending-machine sizes of Lorna Doones and Oreos, 3 Musketeers and M&Ms. Packs of crackers with cheddar cheese and Fritos Corn Chips.

I was making minimum wage, but maximum snackage. I never had to stop at a deli or candy store for the remainder of my high school years. Of course, I did. But I didn't have to! I literally was like a kid in a candy store. What, I gained more weight through high school? To paraphrase Captain Renault, "I am shocked. Shocked to find that uncontrolled eating is going on here!"

By the time I got to college at SUNY Oswego in 1972, I had very little self-esteem and absolutely no self-control. I hadn't had any luck with girls in high school, I didn't feel like I looked all that good and now I was six hours from home in rural upstate New York. But then I found an old, trusted friend.

The cafeteria.

When I found out that I was allowed to eat as much as I wanted at every meal, it was like hitting the lottery! There was unlimited food and I could take whatever I wanted . . . seconds . . . thirds . . . or more. They even had something I'd never seen before: small individual boxes of cereal in a dispenser—all of the cereals I never got to eat as a kid! Hello, my old pal, Tony the Tiger. Yo, Dig 'Em Frog, whassup? Tell Toucan Sam to meet us at my dorm room for a par-tay!!!

To be clear, it wasn't just my poor food choices making me fat. I didn't realize the quantity of food I was consuming either. If I went to McDonald's, it was impossible for me to order a plain cheeseburger and small fries. I had to get two Quarter Pounders with cheese, two large orders of fries and a large vanilla shake.

I know what you're thinking. But at the time, I had no clue. When I got to college I weighed somewhere around two hundred pounds—looking back at it, not a *horrible* weight for a guy my size. Unfortunately, by the end of freshman year, I had gained at least twenty-five pounds. But I always wore loose clothing, primarily flannel shirts and overalls, so despite my weight gain throughout the year, my clothes still fit. Snugger, perhaps, but

••

21

still wearable. By my sophomore year, I had ballooned to nearly two hundred forty pounds. But something was about to change the course of my weight gain and future career, kicking off what would become a never-ending struggle of yo-yo dieting and the battle of the bulge.

• •

CHAPTER TWO

The Fat,
Jolly Weatherman

I never had a desire to be an on-camera television personality so much as an interest in working behind the camera. I wanted to be a producer or a director. After I took my first Television Performance class, the Radio and TV Department chairman, Dr. Lewis O'Donnell, told me I had the perfect face for . . . radio. There was a kid from Long Island in that class. A quiet guy who wanted to do stand-up comedy. Maybe you've heard of him. Jerry Seinfeld? Yeah. He left after sophomore year to go to Queens College and be closer to the stand-up scene in NYC. Imagine what he could've achieved if he had stayed at Oswego for the full four years.

Let's face it. "Doc," as we called Lew O'Donnell, was probably right. In 1974, an overweight black kid with glasses and an

••

23

already receding hairline was not the most likely candidate to be plucked from obscurity and set on the fast track to stardom.

So imagine my surprise when he inexplicably put me up for a job at the end of my sophomore year doing the weekend weather at the local CBS affiliate, WHEN in Syracuse. He happened to work at the station doing a kids' show called *The Magic Toy Shop* and put in a good word for me. I wasn't especially drawn to weather or meteorology, but hey—it was a paying job. Ironically, I had taken a meteorology class for a science requirement, so I reluctantly made an audition tape at school and Doc gave it to the news director, Andy Brigham. In a decision that could have potentially ended his career, Brigham offered me—an over-weight, bespectacled, untried college sophomore—the weekend weather spot, appearing on the six and eleven p.m. news, both Saturdays and Sundays. They must have been pretty desperate to fill the slot to give it to a guy like me.

I was paid ten dollars a newscast. I thought the pay was great, that is until the oil embargo happened and gas went from thirty-seven cents a gallon to a dollar! (Don't you wish those days would come back?) My college was forty miles from Syracuse, so I spent most of what I was making commuting back and forth. I found some people to carpool with, each of us chipping in for gas, and got through the gas spike as best as I could. By this time I was living off campus, so one of the things I did to make ends meet was to eat inexpensive and very fattening food, such as pizza, roast beef or meatball subs from the Oswego Sub Shop.

There was also a place called Cahill's Fish Market that served up the best fried fish and chips, which came in a greasy paper bag. I'd head over there most every Friday night. I wasn't really a drinker in college, so while other guys were getting beer guts,

I was growing mine by eating all of the wrong foods in massive quantities.

Even though my original desire was to work behind the camera, I remember thinking that I might be able to do the weather for a living. Of course, I didn't fit the image of the other anchors at our station. Ron Curtis, the Walter Cronkite of Syracuse, dubbed me "Big Al" because I was definitely a solid dude. (At least it was a slight improvement from Fat Albert, so I didn't really complain!) In the back of my mind, I knew that if I was going to succeed on television, I would have to lose weight. Weight Watchers offered free classes on campus, so I tried their program and lost twenty pounds—only to put the weight right back on as soon as I stopped following their plan. Next, I experimented with all sorts of extreme deprivation diets, which sent my weight yo-yoing back and forth. Up, down, up, down.

By the end of my senior year, I knew I wanted to get out of upstate New York. Although Syracuse and Oswego can be lovely places to live, I wanted to move up to a station in a larger market. In order to do that, I needed to start focusing on my career— which meant really losing some weight.

I received my BA in Communications in 1976, and on the same day married my college girlfriend, Mary Puglisi. I was ready to take on the world! We left Oswego and got an apartment together in Mattydale, just outside of Syracuse. By this time, I'd been promoted from the weekend weatherman to doing two broadcasts a night, five days a week. I wanted to get serious about getting into shape, so I embarked on a diet I'd come up with from my many years of trying—and failing. I ate a bowl of Special K with skim milk and a banana for breakfast, a green salad with a can of tuna on top for lunch and either broiled chicken or fish, a small green salad and some type of steamed vegetable for dinner.

In between the six and eleven o'clock newscasts, I got in my exercise by going to the local YMCA to play in a nightly pickup game of basketball. Over the course of the next six months, I dropped sixty pounds. I looked and felt awesome.

With my new confidence and newly slim frame, I received a job offer from WTTG in Washington, DC. The move would double my salary from twelve thousand dollars a year to twenty-four thousand! In my mind, I'd hit the big time. Washington, DC, is in the top ten television markets and WTTG was the number one ten p.m. news in the region. It turned out that they were the *only* ten p.m. newscast in the region, and hardly anyone tuned in, but I didn't care. In fact, it was actually a blessing in disguise, because I was able to get some much-needed experience without too many people witnessing my mistakes.

There was another, much bigger blessing. And if I hadn't gotten that job, I would've never met the man who, other than my dad, had the biggest influence on my life. In fact, if ever there was a man I consider my second dad, it's Willard Scott.

My mentor, Willard Scott, has been a pioneer in so many ways. He was the original fat, funny weather guy. A native of Alexandria, Virginia, Willard was an NBC page at WRC-TV and was in the control room in Washington, DC, the morning the *Today* show went on the air. He was responsible for connecting Dave Garroway with the meteorologist from the National Weather Bureau, as it was then called, so he could tell Garroway where to draw the fronts, highs, lows and temps on a giant chalkboard map of the United States, live on the air.

After a stint as half of a successful morning radio team, he was Bozo the Clown for the Washington area, then became an announcer on WRC-TV. Eventually, he was the weather guy on WRC's evening newscasts. Willard was the most popular news personality in the history of Washington television. He was also a big guy, over six feet tall and tipping the scales at over two hundred fifty pounds.

A couple of weeks after I started at the station, my phone rang. On the other end was a man speaking with a very thick Southern accent. At first, I thought it was someone playing a joke on me, because he sounded like Foghorn Leghorn.

"Is this Al Roker?" he said.

"Yes, it is."

"Well, this is Willard Scott and I am outside your studio. I'd like to take you to dinner."

I couldn't believe that the most popular television personality in Washington was calling me. Looking back, I think he saw a kindred spirit. It was pretty clear we both liked to eat. So I accepted his invitation on the spot. We went to Alfredo's La Trattoria restaurant and spent hours talking life, careers and oh yeah, a little bit of weather. He was the one who told me always to be myself. "Hey, brother," he would say. "So what if they think you're funny because you're fat. You're the one laughing all the way to the bank!"

And hard as it might be to believe, Willard and I shared something else in common besides our size. We're both really shy and a little anxious when it comes to performing. Willard used to have to, as he put it, "lick a Prozac" to get through a speaking gig. He later publicly admitted he had a problem with alcohol and dealt with that. He also self-medicated with food the same as I did. Eating helped us deal with insecurity and self-doubt. Like second father, like son. For many years he struggled with his weight, knowing that high blood pressure and hypertension were part of his genetic code.

Of course, Willard went on to become the beloved weatherman on the *Today* show for sixteen years and is still on, presenting the hundred-year-old birthdays via a spinning jar of Smucker's strawberry jam. I'm happy to say he's lost weight and splits his time between Florida and New England and, at seventy-six, is probably healthier than he's ever been.

Even though I didn't know it at the time, Willard would play a major role in my future career. And it all started with dinner one night.

Even though I wasn't ready for a city the size of Washington, DC, it was a great learning experience that eventually led me to my first job with NBC in 1978, when I was hired at WKYC-TV in Cleveland. Cleveland is a good-sized Midwestern city that offered a mix of eastern European food, delicious barbecue and hearty Midwestern comfort food—none of which was what the doctor ordered for someone with my proclivity for eating. It was there in Cleveland where I tried my first liquid diet, and in a quest to lose weight and gain viewers I offered myself up as a guinea pig for each new diet that came down the pike. Over the course of five years, viewers watched me yo-yo from two hundred sixty pounds down to one hundred eighty and back up to two hundred forty again—several times. To have that happen on the air was frustrating, even humiliating, to go through this so publicly. Over the long haul, I had no self-control and every one of my viewers knew it. Sadly, I was the last to know. I thought I was aware of my issues, but looking back, I couldn't seem to make anything work. I tried and failed so many times that I became numb to the cycles.

● ●

My (then) wife and I were desperate to get back to the New York area. In one last ditch effort to land a job there, I went on Weight Watchers, and I managed to lose sixty pounds, getting down to a svelte one hundred ninety. Unfortunately, I lost another one hundred ten pounds when my wife decided to leave me. The marriage had been unraveling for some time. The old cliché of growing apart rang true, although I was unaware of it as it happened. Did my weight have something to do with it? I don't know, but it surely didn't help.

Still, after five successful years in Cleveland, and at my fighting weight of one hundred ninety pounds, I was promoted to the network's flagship outlet, WNBC-TV in New York, as a weekend meteorologist. Look out, 'cuz Big Al was coming home and I was about to take a giant bite out of the Big Apple! I was so excited to be in the number-one market in television, and finally on the air somewhere my parents could turn on their television and watch me. Plus I had a great role model in Dr. Frank Field, the well-known and highly popular WNBC meteorologist who reported not only on the weather but also on science and health topics. I figured that with any luck, maybe in five years or so he'd pull back a bit—he had been on the air for five decades!—and I could move to weekdays.

Just one year later, Frank got into a contract dispute with the station. While he, his agent and the station brass haggled, I was suddenly called upon to work seven days a week! For two months, I did two newscasts a day, every day, with only three days off.

Toward the end of this siege, the station's general manager, Bud Carey, sauntered into my office one afternoon. "Good news," Bud said. "We're about to resolve this whole problem with Frank." Whew. What a relief. I was exhausted, and it was no fun to have rumors about Frank swirling around the newsroom all the time. An hour later, Len Berman, who was our local sports-caster at the time, popped his head in and asked, "Did they fire Frank?"

"Huh?" I had no idea what he was talking about. But just then my phone rang. It was my agent telling me I had been offered Frank's job full-time. He was moving to rival WCBS-TV, and I was promoted to Monday through Friday. I was completely shocked I got the job; I had been with the station for only a year and was hardly a household name. Of course I accepted, but then I had a moment of doubt. Maybe I should have turned down the offer; maybe I wasn't ready. So I did what I normally do in a situation like that. I headed down the hall to the NBC cafeteria and got two grilled cheese and bacon sandwiches with French fries, went back to the office, closed the door and said hello to my little friends. By this time I had gained back all of the weight I had lost in Cleveland before starting the job—thanks to snacks like these and the plethora of fantastic restaurants in New York City. For a foodie like me, it was amazing being in New York City—and on television, which gave me access and preferential treatment at some of the best dining spots in the city. And boy, did I take ad-vantage of that. I never said no to a meal—or pushed away the free desserts that seemed to follow my dinners. I was an equal opportunity diner—equally as comfortable at Sylvia's up in Harlem as I was at Pastis downtown in the meatpacking district. So it was no small wonder that within the year I had weather-ballooned up to two hundred forty pounds. My ever more gruel-ing schedule allowed little time for exercise and I certainly didn't do myself any favors by choosing not to make that a priority.

It was around this time I did something I will never forget. I snuck a look at my medical chart. It coldly and dispassionately classified me as "a morbidly obese African American." That was the first time I'd heard the term "morbidly obese." I was in shock at the description. They should have just written, "going to die a fat man."

The coanchor of New York City's highest rated newscast, *Live at Five*, was a man named Jack Cafferty. Jack was and still is a serious newsman. I will never forget the conversation we had as we rode together to the fall preview party for the media, where my promotion to weekday weather guy was going to be announced. Just as we were pulling up to the venue, Jack turned to me and said, "Well, I wish you luck, young man. I would hate to be in your shoes."

"What do you mean?" I honestly didn't know what he was trying to say. Was he commenting on my weight? My inexperience?

"I would hate to be the man that has to follow a legend like Frank Field." That was the last thing he said to me before getting out of the car.

I thought I was going to die.

As it turns out, I didn't die, and in fact, despite my weight, I thrived at WNBC.

A perk of doing the weather on one of the New York stations was that from time to time you got to fill in for the weatherman on your network's morning show: ABC's *Good Morning America*, NBC's *Today* show or CBS's *The Early Show* (or whatever it was called at the time!). The networks dangled that carrot as part of your contract, promising you national exposure a certain number of times a year. When I wasn't filling in, the job would be filled by other weather anchors from around the country. I liked the change and the interaction with the morning anchors, and each time I was asked to come back, I found myself enjoying it more and more. By doing the *Today* show, my reputation was expanding almost as quickly as my waistline.

• •

About two years later, in September 1987, NBC decided to launch a sixth day of the *Today* show, called *Weekend Today*, to air on Sundays, and I was named the weatherman for that show. It was around this time that I was also named Willard Scott's permanent fill-in. My career was really taking off! But it was also the start of an extremely grueling schedule. I was doing the weather during the five, six and eleven news broadcasts Monday through Friday plus *Weekend Today* on Sundays. On the days that I filled in for Willard Scott on the *Today* show, or Joe Witte, the weatherman on *NBC News at Sunrise*, I started my days at four thirty in the morning and went until eleven thirty at night!

Recent studies have shown that a lack of sleep definitely leads to weight gain. Scientists believe sleep deprivation boosts the appetite by increasing the hunger hormone ghrelin and decreasing the full-feeling hormone leptin. When you're exhausted, your body craves food with high fat and sugar content. It's like it knows what it needs to get a jolt of wakefulness, so you grab whatever is in front of you and mindlessly eat until you feel better. But back in those days, no one knew the effects of fatigue on our eating habits.

Of course, even if I'd understood how my lifestyle was contributing to my overeating, I doubt it would have helped. Let's face it, I loved food. And I loved junk food—the junkier the better! I'm talking about Cheetos, potato chips, salty French fries and a burger with a soft, soggy bun, especially White Castle burgers. Those may be the unhealthiest thing on the planet but they sure do taste good. When they're hot and fresh, I could knock down twelve at a time. In my heyday back in Syracuse, I could polish off two twelve-inch meatball subs in one sitting. I also liked anything with high fat and high sugar, from cake to crème brûlée. I wasn't particularly fussy or discriminating and neither was the weight. And man, did I pay the price! Wherever fat could go, it found a resting place in my body, including my double chin, fat ass and big belly.

And yet, in spite of my weight, or because of it (after all, Willard had already blazed the trail for the fat, funny weather guy!), I officially joined *Today* on January 26, 1996, after Willard Scott announced his semiretirement. Getting this job so exceeded my wildest dreams, it almost didn't seem real. Let's face it—if I told you that a bald, overweight black guy from Queens would land one of the biggest jobs on TV, you'd laugh me out of the room. But the fact is, I did get the job, and I was extremely proud.

I've been standing on the sidewalks outside of Studio 1-A ever since. Not every weatherman wants to go outside in the rain to shake hands with whoever shows up, but I actually look forward to it every single day. I've got one of the best jobs in the world and for that, I am tremendously grateful.

CHAPTER THREE

Happy Wife, Happy Life

I met Deborah Roberts for the first time in 1990 when I was working at WNBC. Deborah had come up from Orlando to work in New York, too. She joined NBC News as a general-assignment reporter and later served as a correspondent for *Dateline NBC*. At the time, I was married to my second wife, Alice, and Deborah was seeing someone, so the thought of anything other than friendship never crossed my mind. And let's be honest—I was an overweight slob who never exercised, while she was a size-four workout fanatic and a very attractive woman. Could we be more opposite?

Not long after she got to New York, I was filling in on the *Today* show and she was doing the news. It turned out to be her birthday that day, so I did what anyone would do.

• •

"Happy birthday! Who's taking you to lunch to celebrate?"

She said, "Nobody."

Well, that didn't seem right to me, so I asked if I could take her out to lunch. I thought she was terrific. We talked like old friends for hours. After that, we enjoyed a casual friendship and saw one another from time to time, mostly at work.

Within a year or so, my marriage began to deteriorate. Among other things, Alice was unhappy about my weight, and it was just one issue that was taking its toll on our relationship. I would do my best to diet, but I was on that vicious roller coaster where I would lose forty pounds and then gain back sixty.

I tried everything. During this period, Oprah Winfrey famously lost a ton of weight doing the Optifast liquid diet. I thought, if it's good enough for Oprah, why not me? So I gave it a try. And sure enough, I dropped forty pounds within a few months. And sure enough, within a year, it was all back, plus an extra ten pounds. Just say I told you so.

During that time, NBC News bean counters, in a move to save money, moved the Sunday *Today* show to Washington, DC, so we could piggyback on production costs of a studio that was already in use for *Meet the Press*. Now, on top of working six days a week, I was commuting to DC. On the upside, once I got to Washington, I could order whatever I wanted from room service and self-medicate the pain of my issues with Alice and the world. "Take two cheeseburgers and a side of fries and call me in the morning!" It was a difficult time for both of us and for my then four-year-old daughter, Courtney, and eventually, it helped spell the end of our marriage.

About a year after I met Deborah, Alice and I separated. I moved from our family home in the suburbs into Manhattan to be closer to work, with its crazy hours, but it was really rough being away from Courtney, whom I loved being with every day. Right around this time, NBC News assigned Deborah to our Atlanta bureau, then to Miami. She covered the first Persian Gulf War and the Barcelona Olympics and didn't come back to New York for two years. I was so happy to see her again. I was single, and she was too, so I thought I'd try to woo her. It was time to go big or go home.

Great idea, except we were in what I call the "friend zone." I was smitten with Deborah but she viewed me as her buddy, her pal.

If you have ever been in this situation, you know that it's probably easier to break out of Alcatraz than to get out of the friend zone. Of course, Deborah said she didn't want to "ruin the friendship." How many of us have heard that one before? My real fear was that she wasn't interested in me because I was heavy—that was my usual fallback excuse whenever I didn't get the girl.

As luck would have it, Deborah was being sent on an out-of-town assignment and asked if I would mind looking after her apartment while she was gone—you know, water her plants, grab the mail and stuff like that. I was happy she asked, and more than happy to say yes. This would give me a chance to do a little reconnaissance on her lair and gather some intel.

Now, most guys given this kind of access to a beautiful woman's apartment might have rummaged through her bedroom, looking for lingerie or other personal items.

Not me.

I rummaged through her kitchen. I opened up her refrigerator and found the three main staples of every single woman in New York:

A bottle of champagne.

A jar of mustard.

A slab of half-moldy cheese.

Next, I opened her cabinets and there was nothing but a stack of carryout menus and some stale Carr's Water Crackers.

I opened the oven and there was still cardboard on the racks. What?

It had never been used!

She might as well have stored sweaters in there!

I was utterly amazed. Living like this was so foreign to me! My life was centered around food. I could *never* live with no food in my apartment—not even in New York where you can get everything delivered in thirty minutes or less.

I loved the idea of having a fresh start in someone else's kitchen, especially a woman whose attention I was trying to get. I stocked her refrigerator and shelves with everything I thought she should have. I bought her milk, orange juice, cheese, eggs, butter, coffee, oatmeal, sausage, bread, cold cuts, fresh vegetables and last, but certainly not least, put some Häagen-Dazs ice cream in her freezer. I stocked her pantry with pasta, tomato sauce, beans, rice and basic spices. I even left fresh flowers on the table so she would come back to an apartment that felt a little more like "home."

Okay, I'll admit, it was definitely a "move."

And believe it or not, she fell for it hook, line and sinker.

She took me out to dinner a few days later for my birthday, and we've been together ever since.

Cue the sirens, the floodlights. Release the bloodhounds and the guards. We have an escape from the friend zone!!

Deborah grew up in small-town Georgia in a family of nine kids. They ate a lot of fried foods, and they didn't have a big notion of fitness, but she was blessed with really good genes and

• •

was always in great shape. She was a cheerleader in high school, popular among her peers, and she readily admits she had a tendency to be judgmental of people who are overweight. So it came as a total surprise to her that she'd end up falling for a guy like me.

Being the beautiful woman that she is, Deborah had no problem getting dates, but there was always something wrong with them, or her budding career got in the way because she was always traveling for work. It finally hit her that she had a wonderful guy, a good listener with a big heart, who had a great relationship with his family and embodied the values she had as a small-town Southerner transplanted to New York—and that very lucky man was me.

Somehow, Deborah was able to get past my appearance and saw me for the man I was beneath that thick outer layer. She saw me for myself, and not as the heavy, jolly weatherman everyone else saw.

As our new relationship blossomed, I was inspired to be my best, so I lost ten or fifteen pounds within a month or so of us starting to date. In fact, I made several attempts throughout the courtship to whip myself into shape. But like I had done so many times before, I'd lose the weight and watch it creep back. It was frustrating for both of us. I was trying but still lacked the willpower to simply stop eating everything I wanted whenever I wanted.

Certainly Deborah knew what she was getting herself into because, although I wasn't at my heaviest weight when we started dating, I was certainly up there. Like most couples, we started out in a honeymoon phase, where things were so new and exciting that neither of us focused on the negative. As time went on, though, it became apparent that my weight was a real issue between us. She couldn't wrap her mind around why it was so hard for me to say no to something as simple as fried food or not go for that second, third or fourth roll in the bread basket, never mind just "lose weight" and "keep it off." Deborah and I would go out to dinner and she would give me that look or raise an eyebrow every time I reached for the bread basket. She'd listen to me order and then say, "You know you shouldn't be eating this way." It became an obvious point of tension for us—the eight-hundred-pound gorilla in the room—or three-hundred-pound boyfriend—take your pick. She didn't get it, and never could because she had never struggled with food like I have.

When Deborah looked at me, she saw an accomplished, successful man who was doing so many things right professionally yet was a miserable failure when it came to health and well-being. She told herself that I must have some deeply rooted issues that were making me unhappy, and hoped our new relationship would help make me so happy that I could find a way to resolve whatever it was that drove me to overeat, and lose the weight once and for all. Like most guys, I never really went that deep because as everyone knows, men aren't as analytical about their weight as women. The thought process pretty much looks something like this:

I lost weight, my clothes fit, I'm good.

Or, I gained weight, my clothes don't fit, I'm good. Intellectually, I understood this wasn't really the case—that if I didn't do something about my weight, there would be a price to pay. But like so many guys, I ignored it for as long as I could.

It's not that I didn't want to change—I did. The deeper our relationship got, the more she hoped I'd finally found a place where I felt safe to lose weight and learn to eat healthy. I wish I had, but I simply didn't have the discipline or skill set to make permanent changes yet.

Despite the obvious differences in our lifestyles, we were in love. I wanted to make Deborah my wife, so I planned to propose to her on New Year's Day 1995, and I knew just the place. A year earlier we had done an episode of the *Today* show from the southern rim of the Grand Canyon, and I remember thinking, "This is where I will propose someday." It was the perfect spot.

Deborah and I flew to Phoenix, Arizona, where I was hosting the Fiesta Bowl parade. The following morning, I made Deborah get up early so we could have breakfast and get on the road. The southern rim of the Grand Canyon is a four- or five-hour drive from Phoenix, and I was rushing her along because I wanted to propose at sunset. As luck would have it, Deborah wasn't feeling well that morning. We got into the car, and almost immediately, she wanted to stop.

"We can't stop! We have to keep going!" I was practically frantic, and she had no clue as to why. Naturally, we bickered the whole way because she was feeling sick and I was in a hurry. I wasn't as sympathetic as I usually would be because I was about to propose and didn't want to miss the sunset. Tick tock. I was on a schedule and sunset wasn't going to wait just because Deborah had to go to the potty.

I had made a reservation at the lovely El Tovar Hotel, smack-dab on the southern rim of the Grand Canyon, so we were just a few steps away from my designated spot. One slight problem. It was a balmy 17 degrees outside!! Not exactly conducive to a romantic proposal.

Oops.

I hadn't considered the temperature difference between here

and Phoenix. I know, kind of odd for a weatherman to forget to check the weather! C'mon! I was nervous. It could have happened to anyone!

When we checked into the hotel, they had a roaring fire burning in the lobby. Deborah wanted to sit there and warm up, but I said, "Let's go for a walk!"

"Al, it's freezing outside. Are you crazy?" She wasn't moving.

"Honey, it's sunset at the Grand Canyon—we don't get an opportunity like this every day!"

Reluctantly, she left the warmth of the lobby and we headed out the front door. Suddenly, Deborah stopped in her tracks, whipped around and got right up in my face.

"Wait a second. You're walking me outside to break up with me?!" Panic and indignation fought for control of the woman I love.

"Let's just see the Grand Canyon at sunset," I calmly said.

As we strolled, we came across a group of teenagers who were laughing and drinking a few beers in the exact spot I had chosen to propose. I lingered for a few minutes waiting for them to move on, but they didn't.

Deborah was getting peeved. "Al, I am telling you right now, if we don't turn around and go back to the hotel, I am renting a car and driving back to Phoenix."

Luckily, the teen interlopers moved on and I launched into my well-rehearsed speech about how when we look out into the Grand Canyon, we realize how insignificant we are and how short our time is on earth.

As I looked into her eyes, I realized . . . I am babbling like an idiot. Move it along, fat boy.

"Whatever time we do have, Deborah, I know I want to spend it with someone special." I got down on one bended knee, presented her with a ring and said, "And I would like to spend that time with you. Will you marry me?"

Thankfully, she said yes. In fact, she was pretty relieved. Carl Killingsworth, one of our dear friends, had called earlier to wish us a Happy New Year. When she hung up the phone, she had a terrible scowl on her face.

"What's wrong?" I asked

"Well, *that* was a great phone call. He said, 'Not engaged yet?'" Carl—who was one of the only people on earth who *knew* I was going to propose on New Year's Day—just had to needle her! Great.

You see, several of Deborah's friends had gotten engaged in the past year and she was getting upset that I hadn't yet proposed. Her friends, her sister—even *my* sister—kept egging her on, fueling her already insecure feelings about not getting a ring. No one had my back! I knew I had the best gal in the world whom I didn't want to lose. But I also didn't want to be rushed. I had an elaborate proposal all planned out and I was determined to stick to it. Fortunately, it all worked out. I chose my proposal location wisely. If she hadn't accepted, I assure you, only one of us was coming back from the south rim of the Canyon. Not sayin' who. I'm just sayin'.

We set a wedding date for September of that year. I immediately thought, I have nine months to lose weight. But I didn't. On our wedding day I weighed two hundred eighty pounds, forty pounds *more* than when Deborah and I met. I was disappointed in myself and I think Deborah was, too. All I can say is that the months leading up to the wedding were stress-filled for both of us and my response to stress has always been to eat—a lot.

I remember going to the airport to pick up Deborah's family for the wedding, many of whom had never been to New York before. They showed up with twenty pieces of luggage for six people. (This was long before the airlines charged extra for checked baggage, thank goodness!) Those ninety minutes waiting for all their suitcases were some of the most stressful of my life. I hadn't met most of her family and I wanted to make a good impression. So I smiled, helped gather the bags and loaded them all up in the car like it was no big thing. You see, that's what good husbands (to be) do.

Once Deborah and I said, "I do," I felt light as a feather—forgetting, if only for those few hours at the reception, that I weighed in at almost three hundred pounds. We went to France for our honeymoon, which turned out to be a bit, well, disappointing for Deborah.

Personally I felt great; the wedding had gone off without a hitch and there had been no gunfire or fistfights. But Deborah was suffering from wedding letdown and from a case of, as the French put it, intestinal "balloonments." On top of that, our train from Provence to Paris broke down for several hours, we were attacked by wasps and then Deborah's knee gave out while walking down the stairs of the Eiffel Tower. It wasn't exactly the romantic getaway she had planned. In a lot of our photos, I am grinning like an idiot while she looks like she's barely holding on.

Hey, we were in France and I was enjoying all that France had to offer, including the food and wine. Wait. That didn't help Deb's demeanor either. Oh, well, pass the croissants and foie gras, s'il vous plait.

It was pretty clear that despite Deborah's best efforts to inspire me and lead by example by eating healthy, jogging and working out, I wasn't following suit. When we returned from our honeymoon, she bought me a gym membership at a very exclusive fitness club in New York called Casa, which was located in a brownstone on the Upper East Side. It was small, private and a perfect spot for me to train. I went on their eight-week program called the Body Blast, a cardio-driven workout that incorporated weights and a nutrition plan. I worked out five days a week, and over the course of four months (I did two rounds of the program) I lost a total of sixty pounds!

I was feeling great, so much so that Deborah and I went back to Paris for our one-year anniversary for a second honeymoon do-over. I often look at those photos wishing they were our actual honeymoon shots because we both looked so happy and healthy!

I was in the best shape I'd been in since meeting Deborah, which made our relationship even better. I stuck with the workouts for a while, but a year later the weight started to come back and before I knew it, I was up to two hundred eighty-*five* pounds.

I felt helpless—as if I was watching a slow-motion crash. I knew it was happening, but there was nothing I could do to put the brakes on and stop it. That's when you find yourself in the middle of that vicious cycle that makes you so damn miserable. You console yourself with food, but then that makes you feel bad. So you eat some more . . . and swear you'll never do it again. And then you eat and hide the wrappers because you're worried someone might see them and know you just ate twelve Peppermint Patties and two Quarter Pounders.

It isn't like I was really fooling Deborah. She knew I was sneaking food and hiding things I shouldn't be eating behind boxes and cans in our pantry. And let's face it. If I was really only eating what she saw me eat, I would've weighed around two hundred pounds. She's not stupid.

She could see there was a problem, but she didn't know what

to do about it. And to make matters worse, I wasn't talking to her about how I felt. I was just eating. From Deborah's perspective, food became like a third person in our marriage.

That realization began eating at us both, no pun intended. I resented her criticism—even if she didn't say a word. A glance is all it took to annoy me. Instead of telling Deborah how that raised eyebrow made me feel, I rebelled by eating twice as much just to get back at her. It wasn't very smart because the only person I was truly hurting was me.

Throughout our relationship, my wife has been a great source of support. She has always been somebody who values health and exercise, which is why it was so frustrating for her that she'd want to go for a run and I didn't. There were many years in our marriage where I didn't share that passion with her. We shared our love of television, movies, going out to dinner and eventually our kids, but we had diametrically opposing views on eating and fitness.

Deborah understood that saying something to me about whatever I was eating wasn't the right thing to do, and yet she felt like if she kept quiet, she'd come across as though she didn't care about me. In a way, she took on my food habits as her responsibility, feeling that as my wife she was supposed to help me. Of course, that was nothing but a setup for failure because it wasn't her battle—it was mine. *I had to take responsibility for my actions.*

Me and me alone.

Deborah is one of those people who has a natural governor that tells her when to stop eating. Don't you hate people like her? She enjoys working out—I loathed it. I knew my weight was driving her nuts, and while it bothered me, it didn't bother me enough to make the changes she wanted me to. Didn't she understand? I wasn't fat to spite her. I couldn't control myself. I could feel her frustration, displeasure and disdain, and still it wasn't enough to inspire me to take charge of my weight and break the cycle I'd been living with for so long. The less I did, the angrier she got. She wondered why she should care about me so much when I obviously didn't care about myself.

At my heaviest, I felt less attractive and it was pretty obvious that my wife was feeling exactly the same way. She once told me that her feelings weren't just about my weight—it was about my lack of discipline and low self-esteem. She tried to help me understand that choosing not to lose the weight made her think our relationship wasn't as important to me as food. She thought I was being disrespectful by not doing everything I could to try to make myself more attractive.

Of course, my weight had nothing to do with how I felt about my wife. It had everything to do with how I felt about myself. I used to joke that some people want to see Europe, and I wanted to look down and see . . . my feet. I used to joke that it was a good thing I was a black man. Otherwise I would've never seen Captain Winkie.

I felt so bad about my body that I always wore a T-shirt at the beach and rarely got into the water because I didn't want to take my shirt off. I was pretty sure no one wanted to see me in just a pair of shorts. I was very self-conscious, and never wanted to inflict my body on other people.

When Deborah was pregnant with Leila, our first, I used the pregnancy as a brand-new excuse to eat. If she hadn't been pregnant, I would have found another way to justify my weight gain during that time, but thankfully, I didn't have to. After Leila was born, Deborah breast-fed her for the first year. However, I'd get up for the three a.m. feeding—since I was getting up for the

Today show anyway—so my wife could sleep through the night. I'd grab a bottle of Deborah's pumped breast milk from the fridge wearing nothing but pajama bottoms. One night, as I held Leila in my arms waiting for her bottle to warm up, I suddenly felt a sharp pain in my chest. A heart attack? If only. It was my darling Leila, clamping onto my breast looking for sustenance. It was wrong on so many levels! Getting her to unlatch and take the bottle was no easy task.

"Look what Daddy has!" I said, swinging the baby bottle in front of her so she would take it and let go of my nipple.

It reminded me of a few years earlier, when I'd taken my daughter Courtney on a cruise to Jamaica. She was about six years old. I had my shirt off to go swimming when she turned to me and said, "Daddy, you have breasts!"

"No, honey, Daddy's a man. Men have a chest." I was flustered by her observation.

She looked confused. "See, men have a chest. Women . . . um . . . your mommy has breasts!" I explained.

"But yours are bigger than Mommy's!" And she had a point.

I started my diet the very next day. Of course, that night I ate like a pig to deal with my insecure feelings.

As the years went on, there were times when I was able to get ahold of myself, would start working out and even run a few laps around Central Park with my wife to show her I was trying. Every time I'd drop a few pounds she would just beam. And when that happened, she started to find herself more attracted to me again. There's no shame in that—in fact, it was a great motivator for me because my wife was giving it up more frequently without me having to beg.

Maybe if my wife had withheld sex early in our relationship, I might have lost the weight sooner.

• •

Who knows.

The truth is, probably not. I was too insecure about how I looked and too ashamed to do much about it. I was still a couple of years away from realizing that I couldn't make these changes because of Deborah or my family—but rather because I wanted to for myself. Until I woke up to that unvarnished truth, I was doomed to fail no matter how hard I tried. In the end, we only make permanent changes when we are willing and ready to make them.

CHAPTER FOUR

Let Bypass Be Bygones

In 1999, Deborah did a story for ABC News on Carnie Wilson's gastric bypass surgery. Her frankness put a famous face on a procedure very few people were talking about back then. When Deborah came home, she casually mentioned the story, as though talking about any other interview she does on a regular basis. Except this time, she was talking about something that was very personal—my weight. At this point I weighed about three hundred pounds. At five foot eight, I'm not a particularly tall man, so I had the added disadvantage of having nowhere to hide all of that extra weight. Plain and simple, I was round—really round. But even though I knew I was fat, when Deborah mentioned gastric bypass to me, I shut right down. In my mind, that kind of drastic surgery would mean I was weak; it would be

• •

an admission of failure. Everyone would look at me as a pathetic son of a pup. There was no way I'd ever do it.

And yet, in an act of desperation, I made an appointment anyway, without telling Deborah, with the preeminent gastric bypass surgeon in New York. He explained how he would crack me open from the top of my rib cage to just above my belly button, do the bypass, sew me back up and wait for the result. Oh, and by the way, I would be in the hospital for a week or more and then recuperate at home for another six to eight weeks.

So I would have an excruciatingly painful procedure. Then I would be out of work and off the air for two months, assuming no complications.

Ooooooh. Sign me up. . . . NOT!

I can beat this thing the old-fashioned way: diet and exercise.

Two years later, my patterns of yo-yo dieting hadn't changed a bit. I was still in the high two hundreds and quickly approaching three hundred pounds. It was around this time that Deborah did another gastric bypass story for *20/20*. This time it was an entire family who had gone through gastric bypass surgery together. We sat on the sofa in our town house and watched the piece together. When it was over, my wife turned to me and said, "So, what do you think?"

"About what?" I asked. You see, I wasn't sure if she was asking me about the story or the operation—but, of course, she was talking about the operation.

"No way," I said. And I meant it too. But then I started thinking about my dad and the promise I had made to him on his deathbed just a few weeks earlier. I could hear his voice saying, "Promise me you are going to lose the weight, Al."

It was almost as if he knew how much I had to live for. Because two weeks after we buried my father, we found out we were having another baby.

Isn't *that* the circle of life?

When Deborah and I were married, we knew we wanted to start a family together. I never imagined that Deborah and I would struggle conceiving, but we did. Trying to get pregnant the old-fashioned way, we kept coming up empty. Deborah's ob-gyn suggested we meet with two fertility specialists to assist us in our pursuit.

A little more than a year and a half later, our daughter Leila was born on November 19, 1998. She was named after my maternal grandmother, Leila Smith, who had died November 17, 1974. My grandmother would have liked knowing she had a namesake. Grandma Smith was a warm and loving woman who thoroughly enjoyed life. Her great-granddaughter has brought love and warmth into our lives ever since she took her first breath. The acorn didn't fall far from the tree!

Now, with Deborah pregnant again, it was especially poignant for both of us because we had just buried my father. Deep down, I was hoping for a boy, but I never let on—not even for a second. Still, I thought how nice it would be to honor my dad in the same way we'd honored my grandmother. In all honesty, the real tribute to my dad was to once and for all lose the weight. And this time, I meant losing it and keeping it off for good. Beyond keeping my promise to him, I felt like I was getting to the point where I finally understood that I needed to do this for myself.

I had given the bypass a lot of thought and although I was still on the fence about having the surgery, I was now committed to keeping my promise to my dad. That's when I decided to see two doctors for opinions—Dr. Christine Ren and Dr. Marina Kurian, two New York–based bariatric surgeons dedicated to the treatment of morbidly obese people. In my preliminary research, the thing that caught my eye about these two physicians was that they did the gastric bypass surgery arthroscopically—cutting the hospital stay to a couple of days and the recovery time to somewhere around two weeks—and they both were experienced performing the lap band procedure as well.

I didn't tell Deborah I was going to see the doctors because I didn't want to raise any false hope. I wasn't convinced I was ready to go through with it, and if I changed my mind, I didn't want to feel as if I had to defend my decision. As much as my father was a catalyst, I'd come to the realization that I had to do it because I *wanted* to—not because I said I would.

In the weeks that had passed since my father's death, it had finally sunk in that you can't lose weight for your wife, your mother, your father or anyone else except yourself.

It HAS to be for YOU.

With that in mind, I first met with Dr. Ren, who steered me toward the lap band. A gastric band (commonly known as a lap band) surgical procedure is a purely restrictive approach to reducing the capacity of the stomach. A band is placed around the upper part of the stomach, creating two compartments, one small and one larger, with a narrow passage in between. Because the top compartment is smaller, it takes less food to make you feel full, which naturally decreases your overall food intake; and the narrow passage means it takes longer for your food to be digested, which also helps you feel less hungry. In contrast to gastric bypass surgery, the lap band doesn't alter your digestive system in any way, there are fewer risks and the band can be adjusted according to your weight loss needs.

Another unique feature of the lap band is that it's completely reversible. While that may be appealing for some people, to me, it was actually a drawback. I know myself well enough to understand that if I can get out of something—I will. I was afraid I didn't have the discipline to simply eat less, even if the band made me feel full sooner. Plus, the lap band had a 25 to 30 percent failure rate. Heck, I already had that failure rate on my own.

Next, I met with Dr. Kurian. During our consultation, I noticed a picture in her office of Dr. Ren and Dr. Kurian together!

"Is that Christine Ren?" I asked.

"Yes, we were on vacation together. We're good friends."

Yikes!

It's not that I didn't like Dr. Ren—I did! But suddenly I felt like I was cheating on her with her best friend.

Dr. Kurian instilled a certain fear in me that gastric bypass surgery is not a decision to be taken lightly. And guess what. That's a good thing. It's an extremely serious surgery that even in 2001, after more than two decades in use, still carried a frightening one in two hundred fatality rate. Gastric bypass surgery essentially makes the stomach permanently smaller by dividing it into two distinct compartments and closing them off by a row of staples. That way, food is allowed to enter only the smaller, egg-size compartment. That's right. She was going to take my stomach from the size of a deflated football down to the size of an egg.

"What happens to the larger compartment?" you're wondering. It's still there, just hanging around, but it doesn't see any food.

Dr. Kurian explained that in her surgery she also bypasses a part of the small intestine to ensure that the body absorbs fewer calories and nutrients from whatever food is consumed as an additional way to reduce her patient's weight. As a result, I'd have to take an assortment of vitamins and minerals every day for the rest of my life. Although the surgery has increasingly grown in popularity, it's a drastic measure, only performed on patients who are at least one hundred pounds overweight, about 5 percent of the population of the United States (while two-thirds of the people in the country are classified as overweight). Although the gastric bypass can be reversed, it is rarely done because it carries even greater risk than the original procedure itself.

My medical history made me a very good candidate for the gastric bypass surgery. Even at my worst weight, my blood pressure was never bad and my cholesterol levels were always within the normal range. (My wife has always been fit yet has high cholesterol, so you never know what genetic card you've been dealt until it becomes an issue.) I had no heart problems or diabetes, so despite my size, I was otherwise pretty healthy. But I also knew I had to do something drastic because I'd exhausted every diet alternative known to man.

In addition to trying a liquid diet, over the decades I'd done Atkins, Scarsdale, the Beverly Hills Diet, the Pineapple diet, Weight Watchers, Jenny Craig, Nutrisystem, Sugar Busters, the Carbohydrate Addict's diet and even an occasional barter with God! I knew for sure that surgery was the only option left—and having promised my dad and with a new baby on the way, I had every reason in the world to make it happen.

A couple of days after I met the two doctors, I was walking along Lexington Avenue thinking about going to the Lexington Candy Shop for some rice pudding when I walked past a young woman.

"What, you don't speak?" she said.

I stopped, turned and looked at her, thinking it was either a fan or someone I simply didn't recognize. But then it dawned on me that her voice was very familiar.

"Al, it's me, Molly Goldberg!" She is the daughter of one of Deborah's producers at ABC News, Alan Goldberg. I hadn't seen her for a couple of years.

"Wow! You look great!" I said. And she did. Molly was about one hundred pounds lighter than the last time I had seen her.

We stood on the street and talked for twenty minutes or so, as Molly offered me her condolences on my dad's passing. Without me asking (I am, after all, a gentleman!), she shared with me that she had undergone gastric bypass surgery to lose her weight. She was the first person who had gone through the procedure that I could talk to about it. I asked Molly everything I could think of: about the downtime, about the differences between gastric bypass and the lap band, and so on. She told me about a friend of hers who had the lap band done around the same time she did her gastric bypass—who was also doing well but hadn't lost nearly as much weight—and gave me great tips like hiring someone to help me get dressed and get around for the first two weeks after the surgery.

Seeing Molly that day was the final piece of the puzzle for me. Despite the risks, all indications were pointing me toward the gastric bypass. Once I found out my insurance would cover the operation, it was a pretty easy decision.

"That's it. I have to do this!"

Even though I had had some success losing weight over the years, I finally had to admit that I couldn't beat it on my own. I scheduled my surgery for March 15, 2002. Now I just had to tell Deborah.

In late January, I asked her to come to a doctor's appointment with me because I was seriously considering gastric bypass surgery. (I didn't want her to know I'd already scheduled the procedure until after we all met.) I assured her nothing was wrong and there was no need to worry.

Dr. Kurian explained everything involved in the surgery in clear and precise terms. Remember, my wife is a reporter, so she's not afraid to ask the tough questions. The more Dr. Kurian talked, the more apprehensive Deborah became.

"I don't know if Al needs this. . . ." Much to my surprise, Deborah was trying to talk me out of it. The more she heard about the risks, the deeper reality must have set in.

"You were the one who wanted me to do something!" That was the best comeback I had. I know. It wasn't very strong, but it was all I had.

"You could die from this!" she said.

But I didn't care. I could die if I didn't have the surgery, too.

To be honest, I knew that I couldn't live like this anymore. And I had a lot to live for: Deborah, Courtney and Leila, our new baby-to-be. Mom and my whole family. A terrific career. At that point, I was desperate to do anything I could to stick around.

Once Deborah realized I was committed to doing it, she got behind me 100 percent. She started doing even more research on the procedure and peppered my doctor with her many questions and concerns to make sure we knew every possible risk. I could tell she still had reservations and was really nervous about the risks versus the rewards, but she was still extremely supportive—which I deeply appreciated. I told her I didn't want to tell anyone my plan—not my mom, my siblings, my coworkers, *no one*—just in case I got cold feet and changed my mind or if for some reason the procedure failed—or worse, if *I* failed, because it *is* possible to eat enough to gain weight if you're not extremely careful. I didn't want to end up looking like a coward or, worse, a jerk. And besides, seeing how Deborah reacted to the news, I was pretty sure others would have very strong opinions or similar reactions, too. I didn't want to second-guess my decision and I didn't need anyone telling me horror stories of surgeries gone wrong.

Once I'd made up my mind to have the surgery, I did something I had only dreamed about doing. I began to eat with wild abandon. I felt like a condemned man who knew he only had a short time left. I ate anything and everything that wasn't nailed down. The *Today* show was broadcasting live from Salt Lake City for the 2002 Winter Olympics, so for those two weeks, I pretended that every meal was my last. I had a hotel suite with its own kitchen, which I stocked with Häagen-Dazs ice cream, and where I made thick, gooey grilled cheese and bacon sandwiches, ate steak and onion rings ordered up from room service and enjoyed myself—a lot! Oh yeah, I had one hell of a food fiesta! I was like a whale with plankton—just open your mouth and inhale. I weighed three hundred twenty pounds when I got to Salt Lake and had hit my all-time high of three hundred forty by the time we left. It was nuts and a very foolish way to go out.

It was GREAT!!!! (In the moment—but in the long run, it was a really crazy thing to do!)

I didn't get nervous until the night before the surgery. For whatever reason, I had all but shut the very thought out of my mind. I checked into Lenox Hill Hospital early on that Friday morning in March. I felt like "dead man walking"—a fat dead man walking.

I'd elected to have the procedure done on a Friday because the hospital is less crowded and I'd have the weekend to recuperate peacefully and privately and get out of there before the hustle and bustle began the following week. When we arrived at the hospital, Deborah began asking a bunch of questions, most of which we already had the answers to. I think she was feeling very protective, but she was also scared and trying to regain some sense of control. I just wanted to get the party started. All I could think was, "C'mon! Let's go. Let's get moving!"

To this day I believe the surgery was meant to be. It usually takes three hours to complete, but mine was done in an hour and forty minutes. While I was in recovery, Dr. Kurian explained how well the operation had gone. If everything stayed as is, I could go home by Monday morning. I remember thinking, "This doesn't hurt that bad." It felt like someone punched me in the gut. I was expecting much worse. And there was one change that was apparent almost immediately—I wasn't hungry.

I went home the following Monday. On Molly's advice, I'd hired an aide to help me for two weeks, but on Wednesday, I dismissed her, because I was totally fine. In fact, I was feeling so good that I wanted to go back to work. Deborah said, "I know you had this surgery, but it doesn't seem like you did!" And she was right. My physical recovery was remarkably easy. Now I just had to relearn how to eat.

There is a pretty strict diet anyone who has a gastric bypass must follow for the first eight weeks after surgery. I was told it would take more time to eat my meals, and that I'd likely be eating with more frequency each day than I'd been used to. The diet is necessary to allow the body time to recover from the surgery and to give me time to get used to my much smaller stomach.

There are four stages, and if I followed them, at the end of the eight weeks, I would be able to return to eating many of the foods I ate in the past, but in much smaller portions. Of course, the whole idea is that I would want to make better, healthier choices than the food that put me in the obese category in the first place.

The first stage consists of gelatin and clear liquids for the first twenty-four to forty-eight hours. By the time I left the hospital, I was ready to move into the second stage, where I was allowed to eat baby food, low-sugar protein shakes and strained pureed foods. The basic rule of thumb for this stage is "If you have to chew it, it is not part of stage two." I was told to drink at least thirty-two ounces of liquid each day and sixty grams of protein.

Stage three, which usually starts about two weeks after the surgery, adds soft foods back into the diet, as long as they are high in protein. Despite my doctor's warnings, I actually took my first bites of solid food five days after surgery. I scrambled an egg and ate a quarter of it—if that. I was very careful not to overdo it, because the side effect is throwing up—and man, I hate throwing up. Besides, my stomach was still sore and the mere *thought* of vomiting was enough to make me gag.

The final stage allows you to eat pretty much anything you want, but just a lot less of it. I had to make sure I chewed my food until it was liquid, which took some getting used to. I also had to cut my food into much smaller pieces than I had previously done and limit my sugar and fat intake. Despite my best efforts, there were a few times early on when I ate too fast and vomited. Let me tell you—*that* will teach anyone to slow down!

And then there's dumping.

Okay, if you're squeamish or can't handle talking about poop, just turn the page because I've got to go . . . there. Gastric bypass patients can experience dumping—a syndrome encompassing dizziness, nausea, vomiting and diarrhea—when they eat something that is higher in fat or sugar than is recommended. The body can't break those foods down, so they pass right through and come right out. This "phenomenon" can be terribly embarrassing, and a lesson many patients have to learn the hard way.

On my first day back at work, about ten days postsurgery, one of the producers asked me to do a barbecue segment. Now, everyone knows I love to grill and barbecued food is one of my specialties. Normally, I would have been excited to do the piece. The problem was that no one knew I'd had the surgery and I didn't know the effect a couple of bites of barbecued ribs would have on my body. Before the segment was over, I realized it was a bad move. The second we were off the air, I sidled off to the bathroom.

I know. Bad, right?

But not as bad as one particular day in Washington, DC, that I will never forget.

About a month after my surgery, I was invited to the White House for the President's annual Easter Egg Roll. When you visit the White House, you have to go through security at the east gate. As I made my way through, I thought I was passing a little gas, and then, a little more. No big deal, right?

Wrong.

I wasn't passing gas. When I got inside the White House, I quickly made my way to the men's room, where I had to get rid of my boxer shorts and clean up the best I could without anyone noticing. I was mortified—and petrified—for the rest of the afternoon.

I still hadn't told anyone I'd had the surgery, but I had gone from eating three thousand calories a day to around three hundred, so I was definitely losing weight, and fast. A month after the surgery, I had dropped fifty pounds. I'd gone from three hundred forty pounds to two hundred ninety—a big drop for sure, but let's face it: I was still two ninety!

Even though my weight loss was apparent, no one said a word. Well, Katie Couric kept telling me I looked really good, but no one asked how I was losing the weight. My new look even fooled Deborah one morning, who later told me she had walked past the television set and didn't recognize me!

For all the thought I'd put into taking this drastic step to lose weight, I hadn't accounted for the fact that people might actually notice! I'm not really sure what I was thinking, but after a month or two, there was no mistaking it. I began to get phone calls—questions from everyone from my family to my coworkers asking if everything was all right.

"I'm fine."

"All good."

"Absolutely!"

It was weird because in a sense, I was living a lie—not a bad lie, but I didn't like being untruthful, especially to people who were genuinely concerned about me. I had recently interviewed Dr. Mehmet Oz, who said, "If you want to lose weight in the New Year, be accountable and tell as many people as possible." He was right, but I didn't want to do that. For whatever reason, it was hard for me to tell people and be accountable for my decision, because I thought they would judge me. I had a real fear of being found out.

The clock was ticking and I knew it.

It was around the time of the Easter egg roll that the *Today* show publicist told me she'd just gotten a call from the *National Enquirer* asking if I'd had gastric bypass surgery.

"I am going to blow them off, Al. It's ridiculous," she said.

The jig was up. I couldn't sweep this under the rug or pretend nothing had happened. I had to be accountable, starting right then and there.

As soon as we hung up the phone, I went down to her office and told her the truth. I never intended to put her or anyone else in the position that they were all suddenly in. I had to tell my coworkers, especially my cohosts, before they heard from someone else. I quickly arranged a dinner with Matt Lauer and his wife, Annette, and then told Katie and Ann Curry separately the next day. I apologized for keeping them in the dark and then explained my reasons. They were all extremely supportive. They each said they'd noticed I was losing weight but they thought something was going on with my health and didn't want to invade my privacy until I was ready to share with them whatever was going on. The only person who didn't notice was the one person I suspected would know from the start—the wardrobe stylist for the show. I was losing weight so fast that she could barely keep up with making my clothes fit, and still she said nothing. I'm sure she noticed—I mean, how could she not?—but for whatever reason, she didn't want to pry.

When I stop to ask myself why I was so reluctant to tell people what I'd done, I think the fear was really about people thinking my weight loss was somehow less authentic because I didn't do it the "old-fashioned" way. I actually worried that people would think I'd cheated the system to lose weight. I wasn't necessarily worried about my public image so much as other people seeing the surgery as a cheat. What I eventually realized is that there is no difference between overeating and alcoholism or a chemical dependency. It's a disease. If I had heart disease and underwent bypass surgery for that, no one would think anything of it. For me, a gastric bypass was no different.

● ●

I was also worried because I knew some people wouldn't be happy that I lost weight. Famous or not, you're always going to have doubters, naysayers and saboteurs who want you to stay in your allotted place. It's a pack mentality; when someone's on the verge of making it out, the gang wants to pull him back in. I think this is more prevalent with women who lose weight than it is with men, but you can bet I worried about it nonetheless.

Being in the public eye, I was especially susceptible to this kind of judgment. Not only do people have a tendency to watch your every move, but they're not shy about voicing their opinions. If you gain weight, they talk about it. If you lose weight, they talk about it. If you eat a donut on the street, they yell at you, "Don't eat that!" and so on. And now, everyone would know. I wrote a blog and posted it on the NBC Web site, confirming what the *Enquirer* was about to tell the world. It wasn't easy, but as the old saying goes, "And the truth shall set you free."

As I feared, my dramatic weight loss elicited some less than enthusiastic feedback from some fans of the *Today* show. For whatever reason, they equated my mirth with my girth. I actually had someone come up to me at the gym and say, "You don't want to lose too much weight because that's who you are—you know, the funny, fat weather guy!"

Really?

"No, you have that all wrong. That's *not* who I am. Yeah, I *think* I'm funny, and I *know* I'm fat. But I *don't* think I'm funny *because* I am fat. The two are not connected!"

I want to be clear that I have never publicly recommended bypass surgery and I am not doing that now. I have actually turned down substantial offers from different hospital groups that approached me to be their spokesman for the procedure because it's such a personal choice. Look, it's a very serious decision—

one that cannot be taken lightly because there are great risks involved, and it may not be the answer for everyone. If it is something you might be considering, my suggestion is to do your research and meet at least two or three reputable doctors who regularly perform this type of surgery, not just once in a while.

And remember, whatever problems you had before the surgery, emotional or otherwise, will still be there afterward. A really good surgeon has a therapist on hand to evaluate you over several sessions to make sure you're emotionally ready and have realistic expectations going in. I am eternally grateful that Dr. Kurian requires all of her patients to go to therapy before they have the actual bypass surgery to get a sense of what to expect afterward and to help you realize that whatever issues you have will still be your issues. Losing weight will not take away those problems any more than it will make you more popular, funnier or more successful, or fix your relationship. If you were a miserable fat guy, you will be a miserable thin guy.

RECENT STUDIES HAVE SHOWN THAT AFTER HAVING gastric bypass surgery or a lap band inserted, many people experience what is called "transference," or addiction transfer, which is an unconscious redirection of addiction from one thing to another. According to the study presented at the 2012 Digestive Disease conference in Chicago, "Patients who undergo gastric-bypass surgery are four times more likely to require inpatient care for alcohol abuse than the general population." The study, which followed 12,277 bariatric surgery patients over twenty-five years, also found that gastric-bypass patients were more at risk for abusing alcohol than those who had restrictive procedures, such as banding. In fact, the same study showed that bariatric patients have a two to three times greater chance of moving on to another substance addiction.

Since food is no longer an option for people who elect these operations, new compulsions may replace eating, such as gambling, sex, and excessive drinking. After the surgery, alcohol moves through the small intestine very quickly, which means the feeling of being drunk comes on fast and then quickly dissipates, making it easier to drink more, and more often. One of the most widely publicized cases has been the struggle of singer and talk show host Carnie Wilson, who says she became an alcoholic in order to deal with the stress of not being able to eat as she had in the past. She claims she was consuming an average of twelve martinis a day.

In the end, many people discover that addressing their weight issues was not the cure-all they hoped it would be. Even after considerably reducing their weight, they still had to work on getting to the underlying issues influencing the choices they were making in their lives. Getting thin and healthy is merely the first step in the process of restructuring your life.

••

CHAPTER FIVE

The Indignities of Being Fat

When you've been fat most of your life, when you've lived with that extra weight for so long, it becomes like a second skin . . . albeit a second skin that can be inches thick. But there's always a reason behind the weight, and it isn't just the joy of eating. For me, it became a protective coat. I have always been insecure and I am actually a very shy guy. Although I love talking to people every morning out on the plaza, I don't especially enjoy large crowds. I grew up in a big family, where there were always people around. As a way to get some peace and quiet, I used to love taking our family dog for long walks; it gave me a chance to be by myself. It's one of the reasons I like running so much now—I like the solitude.

I've spent a lot of time asking myself which came first—the chicken or the egg?

Was I heavy because I was shy or was I painfully shy and became heavy as a way to help insulate myself? My weight gave me a barrier that somehow made me feel safe, because I desperately feared rejection. I played the "It's not my fault I'm fat" card a lot as a way of justifying any type of failure.

I honestly don't think my weight held me back professionally but I can't help but wonder: If I did this well being fat, how much better could I have done if I'd been fit? Maybe I'd still be where I am today, which is certainly not a bad place to be, but I haven't achieved every professional goal. One of my goals was to follow in the footsteps of someone like Oprah Winfrey or Regis Philbin and have my own talk show. I actually tried but couldn't get it off the ground. Maybe I was too heavy to lift! I'll just never know if the suits at the networks didn't believe America would embrace a real-life Fat Albert, or they just didn't think I could do it. But I am a realist. I knew the odds were stacked against me back then because of my weight, and now because of my age. Every good-looking young guy out there would have to be snatched up by aliens before I got that shot again. And thank God I wasn't a woman, because there is a terrible double standard in our industry that would never have allowed a three-hundred-forty-pound woman to do the news. If you see a woman that heavy on TV, chances are you're watching *Jerry Springer*, *The Biggest Loser* or some reality show about fat people!

The overweight are a targeted group that suffers day-to-day indignities and discrimination, not to mention inconveniences that are completely self-inflicted. Try being the fat guy getting on a plane, doing your best to squeeze down the narrow aisle knowing every passenger is secretly hoping you're not booked in the seat next to them. As you pass by each row, you can actually see their look of relief that you aren't sitting down. Want to know what's worse than that? Being the fat guy already in the seat hoping the fat guy getting on the plane won't sit next to you because there isn't enough room for two tubbies. Thankfully, I was never so big that I couldn't fit into an airplane seat, but there were many, many times I had to ask for the seat belt extender. I'd always drop the volume of my voice to a whisper as I asked the flight attendant to bring me one. Most of the time, they were very discreet, usually sliding one to me right around the time I was buckling in. I always felt terribly embarrassed by my need to wear the equivalent of two seat belts on a flight.

One time, when I was sitting in the bulkhead, I asked the flight attendant for an extender. She rummaged around in her storage area, then picked up the PA mic and . . . you guessed it . . . called out to her flight attendant buddy in the back, "DO YOU HAVE A SEAT BELT EXTENDER BACK THERE?!?" All righty, then. All I could think was, is there any way to break the window and jump out of the plane? No? Thanks. I guess I'll take that extender now.

Ironically, I never had any issue with car seat belts, although one day Deborah told me she couldn't see any space between my gut and the steering wheel. Yeah, that's not good.

And back in my fat days, the mere idea of buying a lace-up shoe was completely far-fetched for me because I couldn't bend over to tie it. That's why I had more slip-ons and loafers than any other type of shoe.

I remember one time Deborah Norville, who was cohost of the *Today* show at the time, noticed there was something stuck on my shoe. I sat down on the couch, slipped off the shoe, pulled the offending piece of paper away from the sole and then put my shoe back on. She wrinkled her nose and proclaimed, "If you have to sit down to remove your shoe instead of bending over, you have a big problem." Wrong, Blondie. I have three problems. One, I *am* too damn fat. Two, your condescending attitude. And three, how am I gonna walk around after I shove this shoe up your . . . ?

I'm sure Deborah meant nothing by it, but hypersensitivity can go along with excess weight. What seems like a passing comment to most people is a dagger to the heart to a fat person. Odds are that knife won't actually reach the heart because of the excess rolls of fat, but it hurts nonetheless. I actually like Deborah and we see each other from time to time. These days, she's one of the first to compliment me on my newfound health.

One of the worst parts of being heavy was the sensation of everyone staring at me whenever I ate. Not just because they recognized my face—they weren't starstruck so much as judging the food I was about to consume and how much. Here's an interesting truth; not only do people watch you eat when you're fat, they're also fascinated by what you eat if you *used* to be fat. They're not shy about saying, "Are you supposed to be eating that?"

They may say it in an innocent enough way, but all I can think of replying is, "Are you supposed to be rude?" Even though I don't think their intentions are bad, people do have a tendency to say insulting things without ever realizing it!

When you think about it, no one would say something intentionally impolite or make a crass joke to a person who had a physical or mental disability or any other type of affliction. But for reasons I will never understand, they feel perfectly free to make comments and fat jokes as if it were okay—and it's not.

These are just a few examples of the indignities that remind you that you're fat and have no control. It's even worse today than it was ten years ago because of the Internet and social media. Everyone has access to the Internet, so an unflattering photo taken on a beach while I'm on vacation with my family can go viral before I get back to my hotel room. If I were still as large as I was before my bypass surgery, there would be jokes about it all over Twitter and Facebook. But, back then, if someone wanted to make fun of my weight, they pretty much had to do it to my face.

There was one article written about me several years ago I've never forgotten. The writer referred to me as the "corpulent weatherman." For whatever reason, the word "corpulent" made my blood boil. Fat, jolly, rotund, stout, portly and overweight were tolerable adjectives, but for reasons I cannot quite explain, corpulent stung. Now, of course, millions of people on the Internet can say the nastiest things they can think of, and all anonymously, too. I've learned to ignore the chatter, but I will admit to occasionally checking out what people are saying.

Much to my surprise, a lot of people write that they miss the old Al, the "fat Al," the "funnier Al." I think they found the heavier version of me more relatable. I can understand that because there have been many times over the years when I recognize that guy more than this guy.

When NBC was sold to Comcast a few years back, every employee was required to get a new company ID. You had the option of taking a new photo or using the old one. I kept my old picture as a reminder of where I was and where I'm at. I sometimes look at it and think, "Wow!"

If you were to take a walk down the hallway of my production offices, you'd see walls filled with framed articles and photos of me throughout my career. Every size, weight fluctuation and

• •

failure is diligently archived on those office walls. It's sobering to wander along and go back in time—not by date, by weight.

The most startling images of my former self I've had to confront came the morning we celebrated the sixtieth anniversary of the *Today* show. The producers had assembled numerous old clips from throughout the years, and there was a lot of video of me looking really big. Seeing that old footage juxtaposed against my current weight really brought it home. I knew I'd been big, but not *that* big. I was kind of amazed that none of my bosses or coworkers had ever said a thing to me about it back then. Of course, now whenever my *Today* director, Joe Michaels, runs that kind of old footage, he's quick to make a comment or two in our IFBs, the earpieces all of the anchors wear during the broadcast.

"Geeze, look at that video. My God, Al was huge! Oh, wait. Al can hear me, too. Sorry!"

I suppose it somehow feels safe for my friends and colleagues to comment on my size now that I'm not heavy. There must be a natural filter that suddenly disappears, like an on-off switch—the same way as when you break up with someone or get divorced, people come out of the woodwork and say, "I never saw the two of you together" or "I didn't like her anyway."

Really?

Why didn't you say something sooner?

Oh well. Odds are, even if they had, I wouldn't have changed anything. I would have ignored or resented them for telling me how they really felt. I would have let it go in one ear and out the other.

People have asked my advice many times on the right way to approach someone when it comes to weight. Here's the thing. There is no right way. Fat people know they're fat. They know they need to lose weight. When you're buying a size 60 suit and wearing a 56 pant, you know you're fat. There's no fooling yourself or anyone else. So even though you think someone is too heavy, keep your mouth shut; that person already knows. Of course, if he or she asks you point blank if you think they need to lose a few pounds, be honest. (Unless it's your wife. In that case, do what I do and fall into a coughing fit and excuse yourself from the room to get a glass of water and then never come back. Just get in the car and drive—fast and far.)

At the end of the day, it wasn't really my dad begging me to lose weight on his deathbed that was the real catalyst for me. Sure, I worried about roasting in hell if I broke that promise, but it still took me a couple of months to really let it sink in and realize that it was *time*. It wasn't that I was ready to hear what he had to say so much as it was being ready for a change coupled with the fact that I was sick of being so big.

I was ready to do this for myself—there was no other reason; not my promise to my dad, not my wife's begging, not all of the comments I heard from other people about my weight—but because *I* was finally ready.

CHAPTER SIX

Let the Evolution Begin

*"There is no crime in being a big man, it is only a
crime being a big man dressed badly."*
—OLIVER HARDY

Eight months after my surgery, I had lost one hundred pounds
and twenty suit sizes! I gave away all of my size 60 suits and was
wearing an unfathomable size 40. I had genuine excitement at
being able to shop somewhere other than the Rochester Big &
Tall store I'd grown accustomed to. And yet I wasn't quite prepared when the day finally came that Dave Butler, my salesman
of many years, told me he didn't have anything in my size.

"You are beyond me," he said, shaking his head. At my heaviest, I had always been afraid that I'd *gained* so much weight that
Dave wouldn't have my size—a tent maybe, but no suits. But
now I realized I'd *lost* so much weight, they didn't carry my size.
I was no longer a member of the "Big" family (to be certain, I was
never a member of the "Tall!"). As I walked out the door, laughing, I said, "Dave, kiss my skinnier black ass good-bye."

••

When I first started my career in television at WHEN-TV in Syracuse, New York, I worked with Ron Curtis. (Ron was an Italian boy from the south side of Syracuse, but he'd given himself an all-American-sounding name. This was back in 1974, when a broadcaster couldn't have an "ethnic" name.) Ron told me that there are two kinds of men in the world: guys who wore a jacket and tie, and guys who didn't. Ron was the kind who liked to wear a jacket and tie when he was in his office or the newsroom, and I realized so was I. To this day, when I am in my office, if I'm wearing a collared shirt, you can bet I am wearing a tie. I can't even allow myself to loosen it, much less take it off. It's just one of those things that stuck with me all these years.

I have always wanted to look pulled together and wear nice clothes, even if they were super-size. The strangest thing about shopping at a big and tall store is that most of the salesmen are regular sized. They fit fat guys for suits but have no idea what it's like for us. It was secretly humiliating every time I walked through the door, but I fooled myself into thinking it was no big deal because they carried every great designer and fashionable clothes. I was deluding myself that I looked good because I was wearing a Hugo Boss or Zegna suit . . . even if it was a size 60. Any way you slice it, I was still a really fat guy wearing a nice suit.

Matt Lauer and I have always shared a passion for fashion. We can get a little girly when we start talking about shoes or the new fabric swatches from Zegna. We have, on occasion, even worn similar outfits on the air because these days, we shop in the same store. If two women went on the air in the same dress, it would be a fashion disaster, but for whatever reason, no one thinks twice when it's two guys. I remember one particular morning we both showed up wearing the same blue pin-striped shirt, a dark tie and brown shoes. We looked like the Bobbsey Twins—except he has a *little* more hair than I do!

The first time I went shopping with Matt after losing my weight was great! We actually taped it for a segment on the show. Matt took me shopping at a store in Greenwich, Connecticut, called Richard's. He had actually worked there in high school. It's a really phenomenal store owned and run by patriarch Jack Mitchell and various brothers and sons of the Mitchell clan. For the first time in my adult life, I felt like a "normal" person who could shop anywhere I wanted, from the Gap to Richard's and everywhere in between.

I hadn't felt that way in years. Long before my surgery, I occasionally shopped at a store called Wallach's (they've been out of business for a long time now). They carried sizes up to 48, so I could shop there whenever I weighed less than two hundred and fifty pounds. Although not as high-end as Richard's, it was a really nice store; you definitely had to spend some cash to shop there! I bought a gray chalk pin-striped Oxford suit that I absolutely loved. At the time, it was the most expensive suit I owned. But as my weight crept up, I had to move on from Wallach's and go back to shopping at Rochester Big & Tall. It was devastating; no longer being able to shop at Wallach's represented an emotional manifestation of my failure. I wasn't able to control my eating and so I had literally eaten myself out of a store and a wardrobe I loved. Worse than that, I had to pay for a whole new wardrobe because none of my suits fit! (I did hold on to my "skinny" suits for a while, but eventually I knew I wasn't fitting into those suits any time soon.) When you work on television, you can't look like every other guy wearing the same three or four suits over and over. I had to have a stable of ten or twelve to rotate throughout the weeks. And, just in case you're wondering, the network does not pay for my wardrobe because the *Today* show is a news show and not an entertainment show. And the worst part of all? Extra-large clothes actually cost more. I used to refer to this markup as the "fat tax." I guess manufacturers figure they can charge a little extra because the clothes are made with more fabric. I became a devoted Eddie Bauer shopper because it was the only catalogue I received that didn't charge extra for double- and triple-X-size clothing.

When I was heavy, I had to be extra-careful packing for work trips, because if I forgot something, it wasn't like I could run out to the Gap or Target and grab a shirt in my size; frankly, they didn't have it. Today, as America has gotten fatter, the mainstream clothing chains are carrying bigger sizes. Just as I was losing weight, Old Navy started carrying pants up to a size 50.

Great.

Where were you when I needed you?

So as my waistline grew, and I had to free up the closet space for new clothes, I ended up giving away suit after suit to Goodwill, Dress for Success or my church. And all the while, I was constantly worrying whether or not I'd outgrow my new suits, too.

And you know what?

Eventually, I did.

Not only is it emotionally painful to gain weight, it's economically painful, too. I bet every time Dave Butler at Rochester Big & Tall saw me coming he was thinking, "Poor sap. He's baaack! Keep eating, buddy, I work on commission!"

I always wondered if it was coincidence that Rochester Big & Tall is next to Ben Benson's, one of the best steakhouses in Manhattan. They should've put a revolving door between the two businesses to make life easier for their clients. Sadly, Ben Benson's recently closed its doors for good. I wonder if my newfound eating habits led to its demise. We'll never know for sure!

After my surgery, it was a strange feeling to have to start taking my suits in instead of letting them out. A good tailor can take a suit down a couple of sizes, but only once. There's no going back and making them even smaller. So every time I went down a few more sizes, I had to start buying a new wardrobe. It was just as painful on the pocketbook but *much* easier on the psyche than the alternative I'd gotten used to. I was glad to spend money on smaller suits and really grateful to be in a position to donate my suits and know some good would come from it by giving them to an organization called Dress for Success Men, a charity that provides clothes to guys coming out of prison or who are homeless to help them get back on their feet. So often, these guys are big guys like I used to be, and it's hard to find clothes that fit.

I had my surgery more than ten years ago and I am just now getting to a place where I no longer see myself as a fat guy. It had become so much a part of my persona that I hadn't separated how the world saw me from how I still saw myself. Even after I lost one hundred pounds, it took me a long time to stop making fat jokes about myself. I spent so many years of my life using my weight as an excuse:

It was the reason I didn't get a certain job.

It was the reason I couldn't get a certain girl.

It was the reason I wasn't happy.

I had always believed that the best defense is a good offense, so I was always the first to make a joke at my own expense, especially about my weight. I wouldn't let anyone beat me to the punch. I was still doing it when, about a year after the surgery,

Matt Lauer looked at me and said, "You know, you can't really do those jokes anymore." We were on the air at the time, so there was no hiding the truth. I hadn't yet let that person go, but clearly, it was time.

My final "aha" moment came during a photo shoot for the new *Today* show team after Meredith Vieira left the show in 2011. Everything is shot digitally these days, so I was scrolling through the photos on a computer screen and it took me a second to realize it was really me in the pictures.

"Wait a second. . . . I'm thin!"

Deborah once told me that depending on which way I am standing, I look the same size as Matt. While I was flattered by her compliment, he wears a size 36 and I am currently a 42, so I am not buying it, even though I know it was from the heart. Compliments were hard to get used to, but they sure did feel good to hear, and definitely kept me motivated to keep that weight off.

A good friend of mine complimented me on the "skinny" suits I'd been wearing on the air.

"I'd love to wear one," he said, "but I can't get away with the tapered leg like you can."

I had no idea what he was talking about. Then it dawned on me that Frank Gallagi, my terrific salesman at Richard's, had actually gotten away with putting me in a couple of skinny suits. When I first tried them on, it felt like I was wearing spandex. The pants were crawling on me like I was putting on man tights. I'd never worn anything like it, but I liked the way the suits looked, so I bought them without giving it much thought. My mind and body were finally catching up, and that realization has helped me finally come to grips with who I am instead of holding on to who I used to be.

• •

One of the unexpected benefits of losing my weight and keeping it off has been the many great adventures I now get to go on courtesy of the *Today* show. Before my gastric bypass, the idea of zip-lining or exploring the rainforest in the Bellavista Cloud Forest Reserve in Ecuador never crossed my mind. As the token tubby guy, producers used to use my weight as entertainment for the audience—especially during our annual Halloween broadcasts where they paired me with Matt Lauer as Ed Norton and Ralph Cramden, Fred Flintstone and Barney Rubble and Gilligan and the Skipper. But as I started to lose weight, the juxtaposition in size no longer worked. The fat guy/skinny guy joke dissipated faster than my waistline. So they had to come up with other characters for us to play like Dr. Evil and Austin Powers, Batman and Robin, Siegfried and Roy and Clark Kent and Superman. It's been an interesting metamorphosis over the years, one I hope our audience has enjoyed watching as much as we have had fun doing it.

And speaking of fun, since having my bypass surgery, covering the Olympics for NBC and the *Today* show has taken on a whole new meaning for me. Instead of gorging myself in my hotel room like I did just before going under the knife, I now find myself gearing up for Olympic sport demonstrations I never, and I mean never, thought I'd do.

It's become a tradition for Matt and me to learn a new sport at each of the games. In Athens, Greece, we almost drowned trying to compete with the synchronized swimming team—and in Torino, Italy, we risked life and limb when we got on the two-man luge together: I was all gung ho until I found out I would have to shimmy into a sky blue, skintight, one-piece spandex racing suit for the ride. There's no hiding anything in that gear and because it was so cold outside, like any dignified man, I was worried about "shrinkage!" But at least I now understand why women love their Spanx!

There were a couple of minutes of gratuitous posing like two underwear models before Matt and I climbed into the sled. You might think that since a luge is built for speed, the heavier person would lie on the bottom.

No.

In luge, the heavier guy has to lie on top. As if wearing spandex wasn't bad enough, to add insult to injury, I had to lie faceup on top of Matt as we raced down the course. It's a good thing Matt already had two children!

When Matt asked our instructor what he needed to know as the guy on the bottom, he said, "Just follow Al." If the sight of my helmet disappeared from his eye line, that meant we were in big trouble.

Poor Matt.

I was a little nervous when our instructor gave us a push down the icy track. "Have fun!" he said as we quickly headed away from the gate.

Fun?

Oh yeah!

Matt and I whooped, shouted and laughed our rears off the entire way as we bounced off the icy walls on either side of the course. Actually, Matt was screaming like a girl the entire time! I didn't think his voice was capable of getting up into those higher registers. Of course, with me lying on his lap, it wasn't too difficult. We only hit a top speed of twenty-five miles an hour, but with the way the two of us were screaming, you would have thought we were going a thousand miles an hour!

When we finally reached the bottom of the course, Matt and I jumped to our feet, happy to be off one another.

I know how this sounds, but it isn't what you think. Matt and I have had a bromance from the day we met. And because of that, he couldn't wait to tell me what a terrible job I'd done steering us down the course!

"That was the *worst* steering I've ever seen!" he said.

"Oh yeah? How much steering have you seen?" I quickly retorted.

I thought I had done a great job. After all, we got down the course alive and in one piece! Nobody got hurt, so I'd call that a win!

Matt asked, "Would you do it again?"

"Sure I would. Would you?" I said.

"No way. Well . . . maybe one more time. Have *you* learned anything?" Matt asked.

"I learned it's good to be on top!"

By the time we got to the Beijing Olympics, the bar was set pretty high. I was tasked with choosing our next adventure into Olympic competition. I eliminated anything involving guns and shooting right away. (Talk about Hindenburg potential!) Equestrian was out; I'd rather ride an elephant than a horse. And track and field?

Now, that's just laughable.

We settled on rhythmic gymnastics, where the greatest physical danger is death by embarrassment. We got some expert help from Canadian Alexandra Orlando, the only North American to qualify in rhythmic gymnastics. They call her "Alex the Great" in Canada, and after a few hours in the gym, it was easy to see why. She makes twirling those ropes and ribbons and hoops look easy. Trust me. It is not.

After a few hours with Alex the Great, we were "ready" for the big time. Let me tell you, Matt and I put on a performance unlike anything you've ever seen before. In fact, I'm not even going to try to describe it. You'll have to watch with your own eyes on YouTube.

So, what did I learn from this whole experience?

One, I know what it feels like to be a sausage—a feeling I grasped in Torino and perfected in Beijing. Two, rhythmic gymnastics has reinforced my belief that the sports that look the easiest are actually the hardest.

By the time we got to the 2010 Olympics in Vancouver, Canada, the Matt-and-Al gags were getting, like ourselves, a little old—laughable but lame. One of the most popular tourist attractions in Vancouver is a zip line that goes right across a portion of the city. So when the producers heard about it, they decided that Matt, Meredith, Ann and I would have to do it. Over the years, the words "zip it" have had several meanings to me. First, of course, it meant, I'd gotten so fat that I couldn't "zip it." Or, I talked too much and ought to "zip it." So when I found out we were going to zip it in Vancouver, I wasn't exactly sure what that meant.

Perched high above Robson Square in downtown Vancouver is an eighty-foot-high launch tower that seems both daunting and dazzling. When we got to the tower, we were fitted with all of the proper gear, including harnesses, ropes and helmets that we'd need to safely zip across the city. I was cinched in places that weren't very comfortable! To capture every moment, our crack production team attached helmet cams to each of us to give the viewers at home a true bird's-eye view from our perspective.

Everyone was in great spirits until Meredith confessed that she was afraid of heights! Standing at the base of the launch tower seemed like bad timing for this sudden and unexpected admission. I personally think of Meredith as a strong, fearless woman, so I was a little surprised by her growing anxiety. I tried to calm her by reassuring her that if anything happened, she'd likely die of a heart attack long before hitting the ground.

For some reason, that didn't seem to offer her any comfort.

There's no elevator to get to the top, so our first task was to climb several flights of metal stairs. In the old days, I would have been out before we started the trek up. When it was finally my turn, I clipped my hook onto the line and went along for an unforgettable ride!

Brian Williams was on the ground watching each of us go. He had a bullhorn, and as I zipped by over his head, I heard him yell, "Hey, Al, I can see what's happening in your neck of the woods!"

I loved every second of the experience. I felt like I was on top of the world! It was so exhilarating, and something I would never have done before I lost all of my weight, if for no other reason than a fear of snapping the line. Each of us took a second turn, and this time I decided to try an original (albeit unplanned) move I've dubbed the "No hands upside Roker Joker." As I crossed over Brian Williams again, he thanked me for wearing pants!

There haven't been many occasions since my surgery where I wished I still had some of that old weight. For the most part, good riddance. But in 2005, while covering Hurricane Wilma in Naples, Florida, it certainly would have come in handy. Our remote truck operator actually said to me, "Don't you wish you had your weight back?" As I stood outside trying to give my report, one of our field camera guys had to hold on to my legs to brace me against the one-hundred-mile-per-hour winds and torrential rain. If only I had the extra pounds I wouldn't have taken the fall I ended up taking live on the air. To add insult to injury, I'd had back surgery shortly before this, so I wasn't in top form. Add the powerful wind and rain, and it was all but impossible for me to make it through without a spill. Luckily I was okay, but I decided to do the rest of my segments inside that day!

I thought I was the luckiest guy on the planet when I landed my job at the *Today* show in 1996. Little did I know that the greatest job in the world was actually waiting for me—or should I say weighting—because once I shed my excess pounds, a whole new door opened up with opportunities for adventure, thrills and excitement I'd never been able to do as the funny, fat weatherman. I mean, ladies, I was on top of Matt Lauer. The bypass was worth it just to be able to say that in print. Can Ryan Gosling be far behind?

Did someone say Ryan Gosling? Funny you should mention him. The heartthrob was out on the *Today* show plaza last year, promoting his movie *Crazy, Stupid Love* with Emma Stone. In one scene, they reenact the big lift in *Dirty Dancing* in which Patrick Swayze catches Jennifer Grey and spins her around above his head.

I tried to get Ann Curry to run and jump into Ryan's arms but she wouldn't bite. Then to my amazement, Ryan turns to me and says, "Let's do it." I'm thinking, "This is gonna end in tears . . . and quite possibly traction."

It took three tries, but live on the *Today* show, I ran and jumped into Ryan Gosling's waiting arms and . . . he hoisted me up, spun me around and put me down. No way he could've done that a few years ago!

And, on a side note, we've been going steady for more than a year now.

CHAPTER SEVEN

Conquering Your Fear

*T*hroughout my life, food was a coping mechanism for me. If I was upset about something, I would eat. And when I was feeling good, I would eat. If someone made a negative comment about my appearance, I'd get upset and would eat some more. The craziest thing about responding that way is it has no effect on the person who made that stupid remark—he or she is none the wiser whether you eat all of that junk or not. When you reach for that box of Ring Dings or eat that extra-large Payday candy bar, you're only hurting yourself. To overcome this habit—which you likely formed as a response to stress, anger, sadness, insecurity, whatever—is to physically and consciously reset your response to a new, healthier behavior. It's simply reshaping how you think. When X happens, instead of doing Y, I will now do Z.

I am celebrating more than ten years of maintaining a high

level of physical fitness and steady weight—the longest I have gone on a consistent basis. Rather than going on a diet, which at best is a temporary fix, I have embraced a new way of life. That's not to say that if something devastating happened, I wouldn't fall prey to my old habits. In fact, that's exactly what I did after my mom passed away.

From the time I was around thirty years old, my mom had a series of ongoing struggles with her health. Her first major battle was open-heart surgery, in which doctors had to replace one of her valves. Mom was a heavy smoker most of her life—a habit she would end up paying for in many ways. The first time I stopped in to visit her at the hospital after the open-heart surgery, she wasn't in the room. Her roommate signaled to me that she was in the stairwell smoking. When I found her, all I could say is, "Are you insane?"

Mom recovered from her heart surgery, but was soon diagnosed with stage two lung cancer. The doctors had to remove a large chunk of her lung, and she miraculously recovered . . . only to be diagnosed with breast cancer. Thankfully, the doctors caught that in the early stages. It was only toward the end of her life, after she was diagnosed with emphysema, that she finally gave up smoking. But by then, the damage had been done. In mid-2008 she went into the hospital for the last time. It was a painful time for me and I knew that my usual response to this type of emotional pain was to eat.

Ever since my gastric bypass surgery, I was afraid of eating through my new, smaller stomach, and gaining back my weight. It wasn't impossible. In fact, many people do. Every other diet I had been on eventually failed, so I wasn't completely confident that it wouldn't happen this time, too. That fear was definitely one of the reasons I didn't share the surgery publicly until I had to.

Sure enough, when my mom got sick, I used her illness as an excuse to eat—

And eat—

And eat.

My old habits came back with a vengeance.

My mom was in the hospital on Long Island, suffering from acute pancreatitis. Just as I did when my father was dying, I went to work at the *Today* show every morning, and as soon as the show was done, I drove out to be with her for three or four hours. I took up eating in the car, just like I used to, a terrible habit that packed on the pounds as quickly as I could consume them. I found comfort in this old way of life. It was familiar and mindless in every way. By this time, I had figured out which foods I could eat and in what quantities without making myself sick. And nobody could see me eat, so no one would know, right?

Mom was in the hospital around three months, and for three months, I consoled myself with food. It was so hard being stuck between the two places I wanted to be at the same time, feeling guilty for not spending more time with her and not being home with my family enough.

I soon realized my mother was deteriorating so I was spending more and more time at the hospital with my brother and sisters. My routine of good eating and exercise by now had gone out the window. Three months after she entered the hospital my mother, Isabelle Roker, joined her beloved husband and my dad, Al Roker Sr. With her passing, we were all left mourning the loss of this wonderful, warm and feisty woman. And to make matters even worse, I was losing the battle of a hard-earned weight loss. When all was said and done, I had gained forty pounds and it was definitely noticeable.

But the final proof of failure came when I got my fall and winter suits out of storage. They didn't fit.

Shit.

I knew this routine all too well.

The road to failure is paved with good intentions. I knew everything about this process, and I thought I had my stress-eating under control, yet it took only my mother getting sick to trigger those old unhealthy habits—even though I had all of these tools, and for six solid years had been practicing them with good results. You never know what life will throw your way that will become a trigger. It's like an audit from the IRS—you know the possibility is out there but you have no idea when it's coming. And when it does, it can hit you like a ton of bricks!

Once I realized what I had done, falling back into my old ways, it was depressing. I thought I was beyond that. But this time, instead of giving in to it, I used everything I had learned and developed and was determined to fight back. This time it was a battle I wasn't willing to lose.

The unknown can be really scary and that's what makes old habits die hard. Women, especially, may have self-esteem issues and think they don't deserve to be thin so they stop themselves from losing weight out of fear. I'm obviously in touch with my feminine side because I spent years feeling that same way.

Researchers claim a habit can be formed in as little as twenty-one days (sometimes longer). To create a new habit, you have to change your old one. Your body may not want to cooperate, but your mind *can* alter it. The mind is a very powerful machine capable of believing whatever it is we tell it. It doesn't have the ability to differentiate between a real or an imagined thought.

• •

That's why negative mind chatter can be so debilitating. We've all been there. We tell ourselves we're not good enough, thin enough, attractive enough and we believe it! It's not easy but with the right frame of mind, you can change things up.

Thankfully, I now have a new mind-set that makes it a lot harder for me to let myself go. Once you make your mind up that living healthy is something you're doing for yourself and you alone, it doesn't really matter what anyone else says or does. You will stay with your program come hell or high water. You have to get to a place where you believe that no matter what, you are important enough and worth the effort to stay the course. That's what I had to rely on now to get myself back on track. I'd always heard the saying "Nothing tastes as good as skinny feels." I finally understand what that means. When you finally feel great and look great, you'll never want to go back to the old you.

CHAPTER EIGHT

Goin' Clean to Get Lean

At first I tried to rationalize the weight gain; I had lost a hundred pounds from my highest weight, so even gaining forty back meant I was sixty pounds lighter. I kept telling myself that it wasn't horrible. But I knew that forty could become sixty could become eighty, and before I knew it, I might be right back where I started.

Or worse—even heavier than I used to be.

It was a happy coincidence that I got a phone call from Jon Harris, a good buddy of mine from Chicago, who told me that he'd lost a bunch of weight and was feeling like a million bucks.

Jon is one of those guys who after you've met him, you feel like you've known him your whole life. He has the gift of gab and an insatiable thirst for knowing people. He's a combination Good-Time Charlie and the Wedding Singer rolled into one. He's half Jewish and half Irish. I call him the world's tallest Yiddish leprechaun!

I've known Jon for at least twenty years. He is the King of Global Communications. When we first met back in the early nineties, he was working for Pepsi; then he went to an Internet start-up, fitness powerhouse Bally's and finally Hillshire Brands, the international food company. Jon is responsible for touting (and tasting) everything from Sara Lee pound cakes to Jimmy Dean sausage, which proved problematic, given his family history and his love of food.

His dad died very young from a heart attack, and Jon, the father of three young kids, knew he needed to make some changes in his life so he didn't end up the same way. I hadn't seen Jon in a year or so, and because he is such a tall guy, I never really thought of him as heavy, so when he told me he'd lost forty pounds, I didn't expect it to be particularly noticeable. When I saw him a few weeks later, though, I was floored. He looked amazing—fit, trim and healthy.

He explained that he'd gone on a twenty-eight-day detox cleanse created by Melissa Bowman Li, his nutritionist in Chicago.

Now, I had tried my fair share of liquid diets and I knew they were effective but that in the long run they set you up for failure. Eventually you have to go back to eating real food, and when you do, the weight will come right back. So although I was intrigued, I wasn't sold. But then Jon told me that Melissa's cleanse is food based.

Say what?

Yes, food based—as long as it is *clean* food.

Now he had my attention. If I could lose weight and eat, I'm in!

• •

Looking back over the years, it seems that people have fortuitously crossed my path at the exact moment I was ready to hear what they had to say. Just as I ran into Molly Goldberg at the right time after she had her gastric bypass, talking to Jon that day seemed to be the catalyst I'd been waiting for ever since my mom died. I knew I needed to try Melissa's cleanse. I wasn't sure but I was hopeful that I would have the willpower to do it.

I was willing to get on a plane and fly from the Big Apple to the Windy City if it meant finding the magic bullet I'd been searching for my entire life. Of course, there is no such thing as a magic bullet when it comes to weight loss. Every successful "magic bullet" is really the same two basic ingredients: eat less and exercise more. Even the gastric bypass was no "magic bullet." You still have to eat right and exercise or, as I had just discovered, the weight WILL come back.

As luck would have it, Melissa was coming to New York to see some other clients, so we made an appointment to get together in my office. Turns out, she wasn't exactly the woman that I was expecting. In my mind, I'd conjured up a little, old dark-haired Chinese woman who'd somehow stumbled upon a breakthrough while mixing together secret herbs in a back room somewhere. I guess you could say I was stereotyping based on her last name. Boy, did I get it wrong. Or should I say, Oy, did I get it wrong!

You see, Melissa is a young, blond Jewish woman who grew up in the suburbs of Chicago and married her high school sweetheart, a Taiwanese-American named John Li. I had subconsciously taken part in name-cial profiling.

Melissa, a registered dietitian, came up with this detox plan as a way of dealing with her own health issues. All her life she'd struggled with endometriosis, fibromyalgia and later, infertility. In her family history there were strokes, thyroid problems and psoriasis. She witnessed what conventional Western medicine could and couldn't do. After getting her master's in clinical nutrition with a holistic base, and using herself as a human guinea pig, Melissa began experimenting with different combinations of nutrients that naturally boost detoxification in the body. Throughout the process, she learned about different diseases and how each impacted weight loss—a common side effect she consistently found throughout her research.

Melissa's plan is called the PhysioCleanse and Detoxification program. It is a nutrient- and food-based program, making it more effective than a liquid or juice cleanse. As a registered dietitian, she has seen hundreds of clients succeed on her program. The reason it is so successful is because it is not the typical detoxification program where you have to starve yourself, take supplements all day long or live on a total liquid diet. Yes, you will be able to eat delicious meals and snacks throughout the program, but they are "clean" foods (meaning in or as close to their natural state as possible), along with the best quality supplements and great-tasting shakes and smoothies.

The cleanse isn't a weight loss program so much as a way to rid the body of toxicities that build up over time from eating the wrong foods. A healthy body detoxification is about resting, cleaning and nourishing the body from the inside out. Melissa told me the benefits would be highly noticeable positive differences in the skin, eyes, clarity of thought, inflammation, bloating and energy. Losing body fat and weight is an added bonus.

So it wasn't about weight loss so much as eliminating toxins and then feeding the body with healthy nutrients. A lot of toxins are stored in body fat as well as in the brain. When you start releasing these toxins by boosting your normal liver function, weight loss occurs at a faster rate and you are able to release toxins from body fat. Melissa explained that this release is the reason people experience a change to the shape of their body during a detoxification program—especially her cleanse. You lose fat, especially around the middle section where it is distributed for most people. This interabdominal or visceral fat is the hardest to lose but the most important, because it carries many health risks, especially as we get older.

Melissa and I began to talk about the numbers of overweight people in this country, which has steadily been on the rise since the 1980s. The increase in obesity represents the dark side of the overabundance we have in food and food choices. We have become a society that relies on prepackaged, frozen foods to keep our hectic lives more manageable. But are these foods some of the worst culprits stopping you from reaching your weight loss goals?

The answer is most likely yes.

As we spoke, it was the first time I'd embraced the notion of not only changing my diet but changing the *quality* of the food I was eating as well. The concept of *clean eating* dates back to the 1960s, when the natural health food movement looked down on diets that were filled with processed foods—like the ones I was most definitely eating at the time. Clean eating is all about consuming natural, unprocessed foods. This means eating mostly whole grains, fruits, vegetables and lean proteins instead of fast food or highly processed, packaged foods, including man-made sugar, bad fats (hydrogenated, trans-fat), preservatives, white bread, and any other ingredients that are unnecessary. An easy way to remember if a food is clean is: "If man made it, don't eat it."

Some people consider eating whole, unprocessed foods a new

"fad" but it's actually the way we were designed to eat. Highly processed foods are relatively new in human history, and are actually very difficult for our bodies to properly break down. I can remember eating all kinds of foods from soup to TV dinners that were full of preservatives, additives and all sorts of chemicals I could never pronounce. But I can still sing one of their jingles: *How do you handle a hungry man? The Manhandlers!* Amazing, isn't it?

Pick up most anything that comes in a can, box, package or container and look at the list of ingredients. Chances are it's filled with multisyllabic words that describe everything except the soup, cereal or condiment you think is inside. As someone who considers himself to be a real foodie, I often wondered if the flavors I'd grown so accustomed to were from the actual foods I was eating or from the chemicals put into those foods.

So I was attracted to the idea of eating clean, but a little concerned that meals would be boring or tasteless. Not true! You can use almost any spice or seasoning of your choice to liven up your favorite lean proteins. You just have to stick to eating lean meats, and whenever possible choose organic or grass-fed meats, which are usually clean of pesticides, hormones and additives. To keep these choices super clean, Melissa suggested grilling, broiling or steaming the meats rather than frying. If you want to add a side dish, go for whole grains like brown rice or millet over processed grains.

Probably the easiest and most accessible clean foods are fruits and vegetables, which you can eat plenty of when adapting to a clean way of eating. You want to choose fresh, unprocessed foods over their canned or processed counterparts. This means going to the fresh produce section of your local grocery store and not the canned vegetable aisle. We were meant to survive on fresh fruits and vegetables; processing them reduces their nutritional value and fiber content and adds salt, fat, sugar and chemicals. So whenever possible, choose a whole fruit instead of fruit juice. If you must pick a processed vegetable, frozen is always better than canned. But nothing beats fresh.

When it comes to drinks, it's best to avoid sodas and high-calorie, sugary drinks. Remember, clean eating aims to remove added sugars from the diet so these types of drinks will always be poor choices. Sorry, folks. The same holds true for alcoholic beverages. If you want to have a cocktail from time to time, avoid sugary drinks like cosmopolitans, margaritas and mojitos (all faves of mine!) and go for something cleaner such as a vodka soda (not tonic; there's too much sugar in tonic). Drink lots of water or choose decaffeinated, unsweetened tea or juice your own fruits and vegetables without adding any flavorings, including sugars.

Some people who live a clean-eating lifestyle don't eat dairy products, and some eat no animal products at all. But you don't have to give up any group of foods if you don't want to. There are lots of variations to eating clean that boil down to personal taste and ultimately your weight loss goals. For many people, calories are less important because they are eating good quality and healthier food. Melissa assured me that once I started eating clean, it would quickly become a way of life, one that is ultimately better than any diet out there.

Now, this all sounded great in theory, but I needed to see exactly what I was getting myself into before signing on. When it comes to weight loss, my theory is, the simpler, the better. Programs that require you to count points or tally your daily intake with an abacus are too much work for a guy like me. I already went to school and I wasn't about to take on something that required homework. Also, I had no desire to go to weekly meetings or "open up" to a room full of strangers about my "problems."

Melissa gave me the materials to look at as she started explaining how the cleanse works. The first phase is a five-day precleanse meant to prepare your mind, body and kitchen for the detoxification process. It gives you a chance to slowly eliminate things like sugar, caffeine, alcohol, saturated fats and tobacco from your daily routine instead of going cold turkey. Melissa recommends taking magnesium to help get the bowels moving. If you start a detox without a good bowel movement, you can get very backed up or, worse, sick. Although I've never had an issue with healthy bowel movements in my life (the Rokers are world-class when it comes to dropping a load), I understood her rationale. Stuff goes in; stuff's gotta come out. And if you're cleansing, it stands to reason that some *bad* stuff is definitely comin' out. The goal is to get to two or three good poops a day. Melissa told me that most of the e-mails she gets from clients in the beginning phase are about pooping, especially as they are weaning themselves off of caffeine, sugars and alcohol. Poor bastards.

Phase two is the actual twenty-eight-day detoxification. During this phase, you eat nutritious, healthy, clean foods while taking professional-grade dietary supplements and powders to support your colon, liver, gallbladder and kidneys. This phase eliminates toxin-rich and allergenic foods from your daily diet. You replace two meals a day with Melissa's dietary shakes and/or smoothies and eat clean foods for the third, all while hydrating the body by drinking lots of water.

The first week of phase two is really focused on learning all about eating clean combined with Melissa's detox packs, which are individual packets of natural ingredients for liver and gallbladder support, to help start the body in releasing those toxins. The reason she starts the detox this way is to *slowly* get the system used to it while you maintain your regular schedule of work, travel or other obligations. If you started on the cleanse and the shakes at the same time, you wouldn't be able to move more than a few steps away from a bathroom at any given moment. The more I thought about that—what if I was live on the air doing the *Today* show and you know—the more horrified I got. Melissa reassured me that the cleanse works with your life. Most of her clients are very busy professionals, some of whom are on television or travel all the time, and they were able to balance the cleanse with their everyday routine. I would be, too.

What really appealed to me about Melissa's plan was the variety it offered. It's customizable for everyone as long as she can track your progress. If I wanted to eat a little chicken or a cup of vegetables, that would be allowed, while the bulk of the nutrients would come from the smoothies. Finally, toward the end of the twenty-eight days, Melissa slowly backs you down off the routine and into the third phase, which she calls the "post-detox transition."

This phase solidifies your new healthy habits as you transition off the program. If you want to, this is when you can slowly reintroduce the foods that were eliminated during the cleanse and decide which foods you might want to permanently eliminate altogether. For example, now I only eat bread *if it's worth eating*. Plain white dinner rolls are no longer on my list, but a delicious hot slice of sourdough might be. I know now that limiting the amount of gluten I take in is a real key to staying healthy and keeping the bloat down and the weight off. Melissa's approach is to help each of her clients become more aware of the food they eat and what effect each food has on their body. She isn't about three meals and two snacks a day so much as becoming intuitive with your eating. The knowledge and tools you'll learn from this program will allow you to successfully balance your diet and know that you are eating foods that are truly healthy for *you*.

While I came in thinking the cleanse was about weight loss, I came to realize it was about getting healthy once and for all. Up to this point, every diet I had tried was about losing weight. Sure, I knew that losing weight was part of the journey to health, but I had never looked at any program, plan or diet as anything other than a method of weight loss. Melissa's cleanse was a passageway to good health—one I controlled and could totally get behind.

My biggest concern was giving up dinner with my family. I am a guy who enjoys eating a meal at the dinner table with my wife and kids. As a mom herself, Melissa understood, so even though she recommends having the shakes for breakfast and dinner to optimize weight loss, she worked out an adjustment for me so I didn't have to give up an important part of my day.

The other worry I had was not being able to indulge in some of the foods I love most, especially bread, desserts, and candy (my all-time favorite: York Peppermint Patties). What can I say? I love rich foods. Melissa understood my predicament but explained that my cravings were actually driven by the imbalances in my insulin levels, which would spike from eating so much sugar, and then dip. She decided that her first step would be stabilizing my blood sugars by putting me on a low glycemic diet, which meant eating lots of proteins without completely eliminating my carbs. Any change would steer me in the right direction—and this time, I was determined to do things right once and for all.

• •

Melissa and I set a goal to break two hundred pounds. If I could do that, I'd have a little more breathing room if I made a mistake or two along the way—something I was sure I would do.

It was decision time.

Was I in or out?

Oh yeah, I was in . . . *all in.*

For most people, giving up alcohol and caffeine are probably the most challenging parts of starting any cleanse. Lucky for me, neither was a really big deal. I always tell people that I didn't start drinking until I married Deborah and *really* didn't start until we had kids. I am more of a social drinker than a hard drinker. I am not the type of guy who just has to knock back a scotch or a glass of wine after a long hard day. In fact, when I do have a cocktail, I prefer "girly" drinks like a cosmopolitan or a mojito.

As for caffeine, believe it or not, I rarely had it. Despite the ungodly hour I wake up five days a week to do the *Today* show, I never developed much of a coffee habit. I might have an iced decaf every now and then, but it was pretty rare. Giving up caffeine wasn't a real issue for me.

Given my level of hyperactivity, caffeine is not something I need, anyway. I remember about fifteen years ago, when Starbucks first came out with Frappuccinos, I tried one and liked it. There's so much sugar and other stuff in there, you barely taste the coffee! In fact, I liked it so much that I ended up having THREE. That's twelve hundred calories in liquid alone! But even worse, by evening, the caffeine had taken hold. I had never had that much caffeine in one day. I tried to sleep but I felt like I could see through my eyelids. I was like a chipmunk on speed. Never again.

Giving up sugar and gluten, on the other hand, was a bit more of a struggle. But you know what I missed the most? Bananas!

They're a real weakness of mine from when I was a kid and my mom made me her special dessert of bananas, sour cream and sugar. Even though clean eating allows for fruit, on Melissa's cleanse, the only fruit I could eat was berries. I like berries, don't get me wrong, but a bowl of berries pales in comparison to a perfectly ripe banana. And what is it about a banana and the window of ripeness? For about a week, it's a greenish-yellow, then a pale yellow. For roughly seven minutes, it's perfect. Deep yellow, with a dusting of brown freckles. There's just a hint of softness to the flesh. It is ambrosia. The banana is the right combination of sweetness and creaminess. Then . . . BANG . . . it's a brown mushy mess, attracting fruit flies.

I managed to exercise every ounce of self-control I had to plow through. I mean, it was *only* twenty-eight days. If I couldn't stick to the plan for such a short period, what was the point of even trying?

Ten days into my cleanse, I had lost sixteen pounds and was doing great. I had no negative side effects to speak of, and my energy level was through the roof. When Deborah saw the dramatic results in such a short amount of time, she was blown away.

"Let me get this straight. In a week and a half, you've lost sixteen pounds? That's just not right!" she exclaimed.

I tried to explain that men lose weight quicker than women do—but that didn't seem to make her feel any better. There are some people in this world who obsess over gaining a pound or two or even three. I'm not one of those people, but my wife can be. Deborah was born with great genes, but she also works out to keep herself in amazing shape. Unless someone is forcibly stuffing food down Deborah's gullet, I don't think she will ever have a real weight issue. She would never let herself go like that.

First, she takes great pride in how she looks and in being fit. Second, she's on television, and everyone knows the camera adds weight, so she is super aware and conscientious of her weight and appearance. Still, as we age, it is sometimes a little harder to keep off those extra couple of pounds—even if you're hitting the gym hard every single day. This is especially true for women.

Hey, I'm smart enough to know not to offer my wife tips on losing weight because any married man will tell you that's just courting disaster. But around the same time I was doing my first cleanse, Deborah had put on a few pounds, which I will readily admit I liked because she was finally getting a booty! And we're talking a woman who is a size four. She was not a candidate for Weight Watchers.

Well, when Deborah saw how well I was doing, she decided to give it a try, too.

It was a disaster.

About two weeks in, she was absolutely miserable. One day we were in a holistic store in upstate New York, talking to the woman who owns the place about the cleanse. After listening to Deborah complain, she asked, "Why are you making yourself so unhappy?"

Good question!

When we got back in the car, Deborah made an announcement that she was officially going off the cleanse. Our kids actually applauded and said, "Yeah!" If we hadn't been driving, I think they would have given her a standing ovation! She was miserable the entire time, and everyone knows, "If Mama ain't happy, ain't nobody happy!"

Melissa always tells her clients that the first week is the hardest to get through. She describes it as a little bit of abuse before you start to feel really good. Deborah had gotten to thirteen days before giving up. It turns out that the program is more challenging for women, because they have the additional element of balancing their hormones along with their lives.

All in all, I lost twenty-eight pounds in the first twenty-eight days. Most men typically lose somewhere right around twenty pounds, so I guess you could say my results were extraordinary. Maybe it's because I followed the plan *to the letter*. The detox is very structured and easy to follow—it lays out an exact meal plan, which I followed every single day—and that was the secret to my personal success. The amount of weight lost also depends on the amount you have to lose—so I lost more weight in less time because I had a significant amount of weight to lose. Twenty-eight pounds was an awesome kick start. I actually liked the program so much, I extended it for another couple of months so I could lose all of the weight I'd gained since my mom passed away.

One food I developed a tremendous taste for during my cleanse was ginger, which is actually more of a spice than it is a food. The ginger root is an underground stem belonging to the rhizome family. Ginger can be minced, sliced or crystallized to add flavor and heat to food. It contains calcium carbohydrate, dietary fiber, iron, magnesium, manganese, potassium, protein, selenium, sodium, vitamins C, E and B6. Now that's a spice that packs quite a punch!

Ginger has been used since ancient times as a preservative and as a remedy to treat digestive problems, among other health benefits. Didn't you ever wonder why your mom gave you ginger ale when you had an upset stomach as a kid? Turns out that the ginger in the soda helps settle nausea and dizziness and that's why it made you feel better.

I buy several pounds of fresh ginger every week and use it

liberally in my cooking and drinks—especially tea. One of my favorite beverages is GT's Kombucha Gingerade. Its ginger flavor is mild, so sometimes I like to add my own fresh ginger to it as a way to liven it up even more.

By the time I finished my cleanse, I realized there was a whole new world of food out there I'd never even considered. My new, "clean" eating opened the door for me to experiment with all sorts of new spices, herbs and seasonings to bring a little zing to that ordinary baked or grilled chicken, fish and meat. Believe me, I was plenty skeptical that I would enjoy eating clean as much as I did before I tried it, but the truth is, it was so much better. I can actually taste the food I am eating and enjoy the unique flavors I used to cover up with butter, oil, sauces and breading. Now I know that if you've got good quality food, you don't have to kill its flavor by adding sauce or cream. People have only come to expect it because growing up they ate low-quality meat that they had to mask with anything from A.1. to ketchup. Trust me, if I make a rib eye, you won't need to ask for steak sauce.

Life sometimes has a way of making clean eating challenging, but I've gotten to the point where I am drawn to cleaner foods naturally because overall, I feel so much better for it. I'm less bloated, retain less water, digest those foods much more easily than processed food and overall I have more energy. Making this adjustment also had an added bonus: Not only would it help me lose weight, it would add to my odds of keeping that weight off because I would be eating a much healthier diet.

I still go for my old comfort foods from time to time, and when I do, they're an enjoyable treat—something I do on occasion for the holidays or a special celebration. I don't feel the need to have them every day, like I did before. I haven't lost my passion for food. On the contrary, I've rediscovered it—and for the first time ever, I'm enjoying my meals as they were meant to be eaten.

And most important of all, I've learned to identify my triggers that caused me to binge eat in the past and now have the tools to avoid letting it set me back. One of my biggest pitfalls was using travel as an excuse to not eat as well as I do when I am home. When you're on the road, you are not cooking your own meals, and you are mostly at the mercy of others. But if you're serious about your weight loss, you can learn how to avoid those fat traps. For a long time, I viewed eating on the road as if it didn't count, as though the calories I was consuming wouldn't be added to my total. Well, you can go on vacation once or twice a year and get away with a little less discipline, but when you travel for work as much as I do, every bite matters!

Flying is especially tough because you're trapped in an airplane cabin with few food choices. Back in the day I justified ordering an ice-cream sundae at the end of my meal by thinking that if the plane were to go down, I'd regret not having that dessert! While everyone else on the plane would be screaming for their lives, I'd be thinking, "Why did I deprive myself?"

Odds are I am not going down in a plane, so that way of thinking needed to be dealt with. It's nothing but self-destructive to consume three thousand empty calories while being sedentary for five hours!

Flying has now become a welcome respite from my normally frenetic life. Instead of eating, I use my time to catch up on my sleep, movies and favorite TV shows. I love that time because no one can bother me. If I do get hungry, there's usually some kind of salad I can order, but I make sure to ask for it with dressing on the side or none at all. Salad dressing has a whole lot of excess fat and calories. For longer flights, I pack my own meal, usually a salad and some homemade balsamic vinegar dressing that I stash in my plastic baggie with my other mini-liquids you're allowed to carry on. The truth is, unless you're flying a really long distance, if you eat before your flight, you can make it most anywhere without another meal. If you're the kind of person who gets stressed out at the thought of not having something to snack on, pack a bag of almonds or a protein bar to get you through. And always ask yourself whether you are really hungry or just bored. Remember, food is fuel. It's not meant to be a panacea for monotony.

When it comes to being in a hotel, I now travel with a portable blender and my powder packets so I will not be tempted to eat that bagel and cream cheese or pancakes for breakfast. When I know I am going to be someplace for several days, I will ship a box of protein powders, supplements, blender and my personal scale in advance of my arrival. It's like a special travel kit I've put together to ensure my success rather than seal my failure. Oh, look. Aren't I special? Somebody sent me a package. I wonder who it's from? Oh, my favorite person . . . me!

Some people never leave home without their American Express card; for trips longer than a day or two, I never leave home without my scale. I am absolutely addicted to weighing myself! I have to admit that ever since my bypass surgery, I have shared a very special relationship with my scale. Sometimes I think I am more married to my scale than I am to Deborah. I live by the number I wake up to every morning.

I travel with my own scale so I know the numbers are consistent. We've all stepped on the scale at a hotel or someone else's home to find a number either much higher or lower than your scale reads at home. I don't play that game. My scale is an honest gauge of where I am with my weight—the good and the bad of it. Digital scales give you no wiggle room whatsoever. On the old scales, the needle could bounce around and you could play weight roulette with yourself, guessing at how much you weighed and usually picking a lower number than you were. Every fat person reading this book knows that trick—and probably a few more worth mentioning. For example, on certain scales, if you stand closer to the front than the back you will get a different reading. Or you can weigh yourself, without shoes, empty your pockets, or even undress completely—whatever you can think of to lower that number.

Before my bypass, I had stopped getting on the scale altogether, or watching myself on television, for that matter. The fact is, I didn't want to know the truth. I somehow convinced myself that it was because I didn't need to know; my self-image was just fine. But there are two brutal truths I've come to know for sure: first, you can't hide your weight on a scale, and second, you can't hide your weight on camera. Everyone has heard the adage that a television camera adds ten pounds. My theory was that the *Today* show is shot with five cameras, so they must have added fifty pounds!

Deep down, I stopped weighing myself and watching the show because I knew the truth and I didn't like what I was seeing. It was too difficult to face, so I hid my head in the sand and pretended not to care.

My real awakening came six months after my surgery while watching the hospital footage we'd shot as a record of this life-changing event. Although I hadn't planned on it at the time, I ended up using it for a special that was going to air on *Dateline*. We were editing the material when we came across a shot of me walking into the surgical suite in my hospital gown. Right out loud I said, "I am a whale!" Granted, hospital gowns aren't flattering to anyone, but there was no getting around the image flashing on the screen.

How did I ever keep my job?

Or my wife?

I remember thinking, "When did this happen?" By then I had lost a fair amount of weight, so I thought I'd feel safe looking at myself on-screen. It was the first time I had looked at myself at my very worst, and it was devastating.

From that point on, I became utterly obsessed with tracking my weight to purposely pull back the shade and stay out of the dark. For the record, I weigh myself in the buff first thing in the morning when I get up and as the last thing I do at night before going to sleep, so I know exactly how much I really weigh each day. With that image burned into your brain, think about this: The number on the scale can fluctuate up to two pounds in either direction, so I usually take the median as my real weight.

Once I learned to manage the dark holes in my eating, I understood that I could handle them. Chaos happens, but if you plan for the chaos, you can't get derailed. Your healthy lifestyle is a long-term commitment.

What I Eat

Every weekday, I wake up around three fifteen a.m. and knock back a cayenne pepper–lemon tea concoction Melissa has me drink to jump-start my metabolism. I also have a bottle of GT's Gingerade Kombucha, with a lot of freshly chopped ginger mixed in. Peppery and piquant, the tea and kombucha get me moving and sweating. After my seven thirty weather report, I have a protein smoothie for breakfast, and my day is off to the races.

For lunch, I tend to have a salad with lean protein, plus good balsamic vinegar and olive oil. Then I'll have a really sensible meal for dinner. I try to keep my gluten intake to a minimum and focus on eating lean meats like chicken, fish or lamb, again with a salad to ensure that I feel full.

Do I deprive myself? I don't think that I do. I will have a dessert on occasion, but the difference now is that I don't gorge myself. Deborah and I tend to split a dessert, and I find that's enough for me to feel satisfied. Plus I get credit for sharing, and we all know "caring is sharing." (Thanks, Care Bears.) On the weekends, I tend to splurge on breakfast a little more. Maybe some chicken-apple sausage, a couple of hard-boiled eggs, a slice or two of bacon and a gluten-free whole-wheat flax/berry waffle. Not all at once, mind you, but over the course of two days. I am done with deprivation.

Following a routine works well for me, so you will see a lot of repetition in this food diary. You can adapt it to your own needs and desires, loves and lusts. Think of it as your personal food soap opera.

Keep in mind, this is assuming I cook all seven days. Realistically, I cook four or five days a week, but the meals outlined here represent what I might order at a restaurant as well. And when you eat out, be bold. Ask your servers what they can do for you in the kitchen. I find that most chefs are very accommodating if you let them know in advance what your goals are and what you're trying to achieve. And for God's sake, if you're spending the money to go out, by all means enjoy! That's not a license to go hog wild, but it is possible to have a great meal and stay within your guidelines.

Monday

3:15 A.M.

6 oz hot water with lemon juice and ½ tsp cayenne pepper
1 16 oz bottle GT's Gingerade Kombucha with 6 oz chopped ginger

BREAKFAST

1 protein smoothie with 8 oz unsweetened vanilla almond milk and 4 oz frozen mixed berries
1 tbsp almond butter
8 oz water

11 A.M. SNACK

12–18 raw unsalted almonds
8 oz water

LUNCH

mixed greens with tomatoes, balsamic vinegar and extra-virgin olive oil
4 oz grilled shrimp
mixed berries
at least 8 oz water

AFTERNOON SNACK

1 16 oz GT's Gingerade Kombucha with 4 oz chopped ginger
3 popped corn cakes with 2 oz almond butter
8 oz water

DINNER

mixed greens with balsamic vinegar and extra-virgin olive oil
4 oz roasted sweet potatoes with salt, pepper, olive oil and 1 tbsp dark agave syrup
6 oz roasted brussels sprouts
3 baby lamb chops, grilled
mixed berries
8 oz water

EVENING SNACK

1 small bag pop chips
1 16 oz GT's Gingerade Kombucha with 4 oz chopped ginger
8 oz water

Tuesday

3:15 A.M.

6 oz hot water with lemon juice and ½ tsp cayenne pepper
1 16 oz bottle GT's Gingerade Kombucha with 6 oz chopped ginger

BREAKFAST

1 protein smoothie with 8 oz unsweetened vanilla almond milk and 4
oz frozen mixed berries
1 tbsp almond butter
8 oz water

11 A.M. SNACK

3 popped corn cakes
3 oz tuna fish with olive oil
8 oz water

LUNCH

mixed greens with tomatoes, balsamic vinegar and extra-virgin olive
oil
4 oz grilled chicken
mixed berries
at least 8 oz water

AFTERNOON SNACK

1 16 oz GT's Gingerade Kombucha with 4 oz chopped ginger
1 packet Annie Chung's Seaweed snacks
8 oz water

DINNER

mixed greens with balsamic vinegar and extra-virgin olive oil
3 oz wild rice–quinoa mix
6 oz grilled asparagus
6 oz roasted Chilean sea bass
mixed berries
8 oz water

EVENING SNACK

12–16 raw unsalted almonds
1 16 oz GT's Gingerade Kombucha with 4 oz chopped ginger
8 oz water

Wednesday

3:15 A.M.

6 oz hot water with lemon juice and ½ tsp cayenne pepper
1 16 oz bottle GT's Gingerade Kombucha with 6 oz chopped ginger

BREAKFAST

1 protein smoothie with 8 oz unsweetened vanilla almond milk and
4 oz frozen mixed berries
1 tbsp almond butter
8 oz water

11 A.M. SNACK

12–18 raw unsalted almonds
8 oz water

LUNCH

mixed greens with tomatoes, balsamic vinegar and extra-virgin
olive oil
4 oz grilled salmon
mixed berries
at least 8 oz water

AFTERNOON SNACK

1 16 oz GT's Gingerade Kombucha with 4 oz chopped ginger
1 small bag of pop chips
8 oz water

DINNER

mixed greens with balsamic vinegar and extra-virgin olive oil
6 oz sautéed broccoli rabe with olive oil
6 oz roasted cauliflower
3 grilled chicken drumsticks, skin on (Sorry. I like the skin.)
mixed berries
8 oz water

EVENING SNACK

3 popped corn cakes
1 packet Justin's Almond Nut Butter
1 16 oz GT's Gingerade Kombucha with 4 oz chopped ginger
8 oz water

Thursday

3:15 A.M.

6 oz hot water with lemon juice and ½ tsp cayenne pepper
1 16 oz bottle GT's Gingerade Kombucha with 6 oz chopped ginger

BREAKFAST

1 protein smoothie with 8 oz unsweetened vanilla almond milk and
   4 oz frozen mixed berries
1 tbsp almond butter
8 oz water

11 A.M. SNACK

1 packet Justin's Almond Maple Nut Butter
8 oz water

LUNCH

mixed greens with tomatoes, balsamic vinegar and extra-virgin
    olive oil
4 oz canned tuna
mixed berries
at least 8 oz water

AFTERNOON SNACK

1 16 oz GT's Gingerade Kombucha with 4 oz chopped ginger
3 popped corn cakes with 2 oz almond butter
8 oz water

DINNER

mixed greens with balsamic vinegar and extra-virgin olive oil
6 oz grilled zucchini
4 oz steamed wild rice
6 oz grilled duck breast with balsamic glaze
mixed berries
8 oz water

EVENING SNACK

12–16 raw unsalted almonds
1 16 oz GT's Gingerade Kombucha with 4 oz chopped ginger
8 oz water

Friday

3:15 A.M.

6 oz hot water with lemon juice and ½ tsp cayenne pepper
1 16 oz bottle GT's Gingerade Kombucha with 6 oz chopped ginger

BREAKFAST

1 protein smoothie with 8 oz unsweetened vanilla almond milk and
    4 oz frozen mixed berries
1 tbsp almond butter
8 oz water

11 A.M. SNACK

12–18 raw unsalted almonds
8 oz water

LUNCH

mixed greens with tomatoes, balsamic vinegar and extra-virgin
    olive oil
4 oz grilled chicken breast
mixed berries
at least 8 oz water

AFTERNOON SNACK

1 16 oz GT's Gingerade Kombucha with 4 oz chopped ginger
3 popped corn cakes with 2 oz almond butter
8 oz water

DINNER

mixed greens with balsamic vinegar and extra-virgin olive oil
6 oz steamed broccoli
4 oz roasted butternut squash with olive oil, salt, pepper and dark
agave syrup
1 6 oz ground lamb patty, grilled
mixed berries
8 oz water

EVENING SNACK

3 caramel popped corn cakes
1 16 oz GT's Gingerade Kombucha with 4 oz chopped ginger
8 oz water

Saturday

7:30 A.M.

6 oz hot water with lemon juice and ½ tsp cayenne pepper
1 16 oz bottle GT's Gingerade Kombucha with 6 oz chopped ginger

BREAKFAST

2 chicken-apple sausage links
2 hard-boiled eggs
8 oz water

11 A.M. SNACK

1 packet Justin's Almond Maple Nut Butter
8 oz water

LUNCH

mixed greens with tomatoes, balsamic vinegar and extra-virgin
olive oil
4–6 oz lean turkey breast cold cuts, rolled up
mixed berries
at least 8 oz water

AFTERNOON SNACK

1 16 oz GT's Gingerade Kombucha with 4 oz chopped ginger
3 popped corn cakes with 2 oz almond butter
8 oz water

DINNER

mixed greens with balsamic vinegar and extra-virgin olive oil
6 oz grilled corn, grilled avocado and tomato salad
4 oz grilled asparagus
2 grilled sea bass fish tacos with corn tortillas
mixed berries
8 oz water

EVENING SNACK

12–16 raw unsalted almonds
1 16 oz GT's Gingerade Kombucha with 4 oz chopped ginger
8 oz water

Sunday

7:00 A.M.

6 oz hot water with lemon juice and ½ tsp cayenne pepper
1 16 oz bottle GT's Gingerade Kombucha with 6 oz chopped ginger

BREAKFAST

1 gluten-free whole-wheat flax/berry waffle
2 chicken-apple sausage links
8 oz water

11 A.M. SNACK

12–18 raw unsalted almonds
8 oz water

LUNCH

mixed greens with tomatoes, balsamic vinegar and extra-virgin olive oil
4 oz grilled shrimp
mixed berries
at least 8 oz water

AFTERNOON SNACK

1 16 oz GT's Gingerade Kombucha with 4 oz chopped ginger
1 packet Justin's Maple Almond Nut Butter
8 oz water

DINNER

mixed greens with balsamic vinegar and extra-virgin olive oil
6 oz grilled zucchini
4 oz roasted sweet potatoes with olive oil and 1 tbsp duck fat
6 oz grilled duck breast with balsamic glaze
mixed berries
8 oz water

EVENING SNACK

12–16 raw unsalted almonds
1 16 oz GT's Gingerade Kombucha with 4 oz chopped ginger
8 oz water

PhysioSlow 3-Day Workout

Monday (Machines)

leg press
compound row
chest press
overhead press
lat pull down
forearm plank—30 seconds
stretch

Wednesday (Free Weights)

lateral shoulder raise
front shoulder raise—straight arm
tricep dips (on bench)
chest flies (on stability ball)
stability ball ab crunches
supermans (prone arm/leg raises)
stretch

Friday (Machines)

lat press down—abs
back extension
hamstring curl
hip abduction
neck extension
ab roll-out with wheel
stretch

YOU SHOULD CONSULT WITH A HEALTH CARE PROFESSIONAL BEFORE STARTING ANY DIET, EXERCISE AND/OR SUPPLEMENT PROGRAM.

CHAPTER NINE

Slow and Steady
Wins the Race

People always ask me what the secret to permanent weight loss is.

My answer is simple: Eat less, exercise more.

I know, easy advice to give, but much—*much*—harder to take.

In 2010, on average, one in three adults who had seen a physician had been advised to begin or continue to do exercise or physical activity. Before my gastric bypass surgery, my history of working out was pretty much a chart of fits and starts. I'd join a gym with the best of intentions, go a few days a week for a couple of months, and then I'd lapse. I was part of the business model most gyms build their profits on—the guy who pays and never goes. If everyone who had a membership to your gym actually showed up, they couldn't possibly accommodate them.

They bet on people not showing up—and in racing terms, I was a sure thing. The truth is, I didn't enjoy working out—never. I still don't.

I'm frequently asked what my favorite part of working out is. My answer?

Saying good-bye!

Before my gastric bypass, the longest I'd ever stuck with a workout was the six months I did the Body Blast after Deborah and I got married. After my bypass, I discovered a Sports Club/ LA near the *Today* show studio where I could exercise at four thirty in the morning. Actually, I'd show up around four fifteen. The gym wasn't even open, but the cleaning crew was there, the doors were open and they never said I couldn't come in. For about thirty minutes, I had the entire place to myself. By five a.m., thirty or forty people would be scattered around, mostly Wall Street types, who were always competing to see who could lift more weight. Let's be clear, I was never a part of those contests. I did my workout, which was a little walking on the treadmill and lifting a few weights, and I was out of there.

I am truly one of those guys who needs someone to tell me what to do in the gym. I will never push myself in the same way a personal trainer pushes me. When I work out on my own, I go through the motions, I'll put in the time, but I might do half as many reps or a third of the sit-ups I'd do if I were working with a trainer. Knowing that about myself, I asked Melissa's advice on how I should exercise while doing her cleanse.

She turned me on to a new type of workout called the "Slow Method," which guys like Brad Pitt and Kevin Bacon use to get into shape. Well, hey, if it's good enough for those two guys, I figured it's got to work for a schlub like me!

The slow method is a highly specialized form of strength

training for thirty minutes just two or three times a week. Melissa described the workouts as short but intense. Hmm, just like me. A single repetition takes around twenty seconds to lift and lower the weights, and you should be able to do only six to eight reps before your muscles are completely fatigued. With this slow lifting, you're using only the strength of your muscles to move the weights, rather than momentum and acceleration. The slow speed and intensity safely and effectively build more lean muscle mass than a typical workout.

The slow method was created by Ken Hutchins at the University of Florida School of Medicine in 1982. Ken was strength-training a group of elderly women diagnosed with osteoporosis when he discovered that slowing down the movement of lifting and lowering the weight allowed these women to train more safely. The women were frail and he was worried about someone getting hurt. Not only did the slow lifting increase their bone density; it also increased their lean body mass. The results were so powerful that Ken applied the same techniques to other people he trained, achieving the exact same results. Now I have the strength and stamina of an elderly woman. Yes!!!

According to Melissa, one of the greatest misconceptions people have about working out is that more is better. That's never been my problem. My problem? I believe *less* is *better*— and *nothing* is *best*. Granted, I realize that's wrong, but we all come to the destination via different paths . . . grasshopper.

I suppose the debate about quality versus quantity will never end because everyone has a personal style. However, exercise physiologists and researchers have shown that long workouts that require intense energy expenditure are the least effective way to get fit and often lead to injuries or plain burnout. Melissa explained that the effectiveness of any exercise program is determined by the intensity of the activity and the amount of time the body needs to recover.

The goal of a slow cadence workout is to bring the muscles to exhaustion; if the goal of true muscular exhaustion is met, an extended recovery period is critical to allow the repair of the muscle through a process known as "super compensation." It's during this recovery time that the real growth of muscle takes place; that's why you can't do the super slow workout more than a couple of days a week. I know lots of people who go to the gym five days a week but never look any better for their efforts. They don't get the results they're seeking because their muscles never get to a point of total failure. Their type of working out is more for maintenance than it is effective body sculpting.

The PhysioSlow method targets the body's major muscles, called skeletal muscles. These are the body's engine. They produce more heat, consume more calories, and receive more blood flow than any of the other muscles in the body. You use as much weight as you can lift six or eight times within a few minutes; at that point, your muscle will be completely exhausted, or failed. In this case, failure is good. It's what induces the muscle to grow bigger and stronger.

The slow method workout is perfect for someone who does not like to work out, who doesn't have a lot of time and needs to lose weight. It's also an ideal workout for anyone with tendon or ligament injuries; those don't strengthen like muscles do. Our muscles are meant to tear and repair—that's how muscle gets built. Plus, shorter and more intense workouts put less stress on the joints.

Since Melissa lived in Chicago, she researched and found a highly skilled certified personal trainer in New York City, Patricia

Whitcas, who is proficient in this method of working out. Patricia is a certified spinning and Pilates instructor, too. She also makes her own clothes and has a lovely singing voice. People like her make me sick. Seriously, Patricia is the best advertisement for working out. She is a petite blonde whose looks belie her age.

The first gym we used was a very Bauhaus-looking place, with all the original equipment developed by Ken Hutchins in 1982. It had metal slabs, rivets, cranks and an airline-like seat belt used for safety straps. It looked like Frankenstein's laboratory. There was nothing digital or modern about it. The first time I saw the equipment, I thought, "Wow, this is pretty old school."

The owner of the gym had bought the equipment brand-new and hadn't upgraded it since. In fact, he kind of looked like he hadn't changed much since 1982 either! He had a big bushy mustache and Marty Feldman eyes, was barely five feet tall and wore tiny polyester shorts. He even had a framed picture of himself with Arnold Schwarzenegger on the wall taken way back in the day. There was another character in the gym, a little old man who came in from time to time to do the books.

"Who is that guy?" I asked Patricia one day.

"That's his mother!" she said.

Ooh. Awkward.

The draw of the slow method workout for me was obvious: You could get my exercise in in around thirty minutes. Theoretically, you can even do it in your street clothes. Since it's not a cardio workout, you're not likely to sweat. I'd often see businessmen in suits and women in skirts and heels working out. Me, I sweat standing still, so I always change into gym clothes.

Patricia usually has me do five exercises, sometimes only working the upper body, sometimes the lower body, and sometimes both. We always end with about ten minutes of mat work, usually focusing on the core, and then a final stretch. That is by far the most enjoyable part of our workout. Believe it or not, I'm really flexible, especially for a guy who carried around so much extra weight for all of those years.

Patricia and I lasted about a year at the first gym before we found a place called Transform Fitness. It's a relatively small facility with the modern versions of the equipment needed for the slow method. The new stuff is streamlined, taking up a fraction of the space the old-style equipment does. This gym also has a yoga area, so Patricia can incorporate her other specialties into our workouts, too.

She doesn't think I know what she's up to, but rest assured, I am aware when she has me working my core. Every single session she has me doing planks, an abdominal exercise that helps strengthen the core and stability—and I'd rather walk the plank than do a plank. I hate them, especially when Patricia makes me start lifting a leg while holding my body weight on nothing but my forearms.

"Lift your leg.

"Now both legs.

"Now balance on your elbows.

"Now wave hello. . . ."

I hate every variation she can think of!

Just when I think I'm doing well, Patricia comes up with yet another way to torture me during our workouts. Why not throw waterboarding in there, too?

The truth is, my work with Patricia is now the longest relationship I've ever had with a personal trainer, and this is the longest I've ever stayed with a fitness routine. I may not love it, but I love the results. I don't think I could ever go back to any

••

other type of exercise because the slow method is so efficient and effective.

Now, my wife works out with a trainer named Don Scott, a compact and lean guy who is a very good trainer. The biggest difference between Don and Patricia is that Don is not human. Don is a Cyborg. Don only eats when he has to. There is no enjoyment or interest whatsoever in food. I'm not even sure he engages in anything for fun! He is all about training and fitness. Even though he is a big movie buff, I am positive he never eats popcorn. The only thing I have ever seen Don eat is something he gets at Whole Foods that bears no resemblance to anything human beings would eat. It's a packet of "greens" you pour in a glass and mix with water. It looks like water and moss put in a blender. There's also a protein bar he sometimes eats that says it's "chocolate." I have never seen chocolate so green! I almost did a Danny Thomas spit take when he made me try a bite.

Which is why I get along so well with Patricia. She eats and enjoys food like a normal person. I'm not a machine. I'm a human—which means I will make mistakes from time to time. Patricia doesn't beat me up or make me feel bad about myself for being fallible. While I appreciate her qualifications as a trainer, what keeps me working out with Patricia is the rapport we've built. You feel vulnerable in the gym, and she's someone I've come to trust. Plus she never lets me get bored and is always full of surprises. Sometimes I like them, and other times, not so much. But training with Patricia is like playing with a jack-in-the-box . . . a jack-in-the-box with a killer body and a Marquis de Sade talent for changing your routine when you least expect it.

For me, the slow method makes it easier to keep up my fitness routine whether I'm traveling or just can't make it to the gym. Once you master the routine, you can actually do the workout anywhere and still get results. You don't need a lot of room—just some free weights or resistance bands.

A good fitness routine comes down to having the right mindset. It's a psychological thing more than a physical thing; just like losing weight, to get the most out of your training, you need to be ready for it. And when you make that commitment, it's a complete lifestyle decision to find a new balance between nutrition and exercise that works for you. No one is telling you not to enjoy yourself. It's about incorporating fitness into your life and knowing that you need to do it. I am 100 percent committed to my health and fitness. I don't have time to waste an hour just going through the motions. I want to get my workout in and move on with my day, making sure I choose the right foods along the way.

Since starting the slow method training, I have gotten a lot stronger in my body and my core, my balance is better and for the first time in my life, I am committed to physical fitness. If I backslide with my food, I know I can get back within a week or so by hitting the gym hard and training with Patricia. I might protest the entire time, but I never miss a session because I know I need to do it. I sometimes wish Patricia would cancel on me or show up late—just once!—but she won't—not ever. Patricia once told me that her only clients more committed to their workouts than me are her brides-to-be—and they're temporary! They're only there to fit into a dress in four weeks.

Me?

I'm in it for life!

Slow Strength Training Overview

The following is a quick overview of the Slow Method Training program Melissa wants her clients to do. She built an entire studio dedicated to the Slow Method workout. If you're interested, find an experienced professional who is certified in this type of workout to help teach you the proper form and safety for your best results.

When properly performed, Slow Strength Training can deliver significant improvements in muscular strength, size, endurance, bone strength, cardiovascular efficiency, flexibility and body composition. However, when improperly performed, it can produce injury. The prevention of injury during exercise is just as important as stimulating the production of physical improvements. Although your personal trainer will be closely monitoring your exercise, and coach you through each exercise, it is critical that you are familiar with the safety considerations as well.

There are several performance and safety considerations which must be observed to maximize results and to reduce the risk of injury:

1. *What is PhysioSlow Strength Training Method?*

➤ PhysioSlow Strength Training is both safe and highly effective. It is a total body, thirty-minute workout that only needs to be performed twice a week for optimal results. It is done with a certified PhysioSlow personal trainer on our specialized slow method equipment. Each routine includes eight to eleven exercises. PhysioSlow Strength Training works all major muscle groups, strengthens bones and increases cardiovascular function.

➤ Each exercise is performed using extremely slow movements. A single repetition takes about twenty seconds. This eliminates momentum and acceleration, which makes it possible to completely load the muscles that are being worked. The muscles are then able to go to complete exhaustion within two minutes of each exercise. As a result, force is minimized to the tendons and joints, while targeting strength and growth to the muscles.

2. Proper Form and Customized Equipment Settings

➤ Pay close attention to proper body positioning, as well as alignment in single movement exercises. This is a good excuse to check yourself out in the mirror. Damn. You look good!

➤ While learning and practicing a new exercise, your trainer will select a weight that you can easily handle while monitoring your form and instructing you on how to perform the exercise.

➤ Your trainer will also need to determine your customized machine settings based on your body, range of motion and any limitations. Make a lot of noise and maybe he/she will have pity on you and lower the weights.

➤ Your goal during the first few workouts is to learn the proper form on each exercise and concentrate on the target muscles at work, while breathing properly. After you have achieved a sufficient level of proficiency in the exercise, your trainer will increase the weights gradually over the course of several workouts until the appropriate rep time is achieved. When they start increasing the weight, select creative curses to hurl in their general direction.

3. Slow and Controlled Speed

➤ Injury results when a tissue is exposed to a force that exceeds its structural strength. Slower repetition speeds expose the body to less force, decreasing the risk of injury.

➤ To minimize the amount of force the body is exposed to during an exercise, move slowly while raising and lowering the weight, and perform the turnarounds (the reversal of direction at the start and end of each movement) in a smooth and controlled manner. Attempt to barely move at the start of each repetition, and then move just slowly enough to avoid using momentum to help lift the weight. Don't yank, jerk, heave, reload, or bounce out of the starting position. (The same advice applies to sex.) Take your time and concentrate on contracting the target muscles over the full range of motion.

➤ When it seems almost impossible to produce any further movement against the resistance, do not sacrifice form for the sake of completing the repetition. We're talking weights here, not pooping. Concentrate on contracting the target muscles as hard as you can and try to keep the resistance moving, even if it seems to barely move at all. Once you have achieved muscular exhaustion, and positive movement ceases, your trainer will motivate you to hold the position for ten more seconds and then tell you to slowly set down the weight.

4. Breathing

➤ Breathing is good. Not breathing will lead to trouble.

➤ It is very important never to force air against a closed glottis (throat), grunt or restrict your breathing with your teeth or lips during exercise. This is called Valsalva. Even though it sounds like a character from *Goodfellas*, Valsalva dramatically raises your blood pressure.

➤ Take big, deep, full breaths that will oxygenate your muscles and produce the most efficient workout.

➤ It is also necessary to breathe continuously during exercise, in a relaxed and natural manner. It is preferable to breathe through the mouth, with the mouth wide open. Do not purse your lips as you exhale, as this increases the amount of force required to expel the air from the lungs, increasing intra-abdominal and thoracic pressure, and thus blood pressure. And it makes you look like you're whistling silently. Not a good look.

5. *Proper Positioning and Stabilization of the Head and Neck*

➤ Your head and neck musculature are under load, either directly or indirectly, during most exercises. To decrease the risk of neck strain or headache, it is necessary to minimize tension in this area when performing exercises for other areas of the body. This can be accomplished by maintaining a relaxed and neutral position of the head and neck. The ideal head and neck position relative to the body differs slightly between exercises, but generally consists of the head facing straight forward, with the neck slightly flexed and the chin about fist-distance from the sternum.

➤ During exercises where the back of the head is resting on a seat, bench, or head support, it is essential that you do not push back with the head, increasing tension in the neck.

➤ When on a machine, do not make eye contact with your trainer; position your head facing straight forward. In fact, never make eye contact with your trainer. Ignore him/her, pack your bag, walk out and never return. Kidding.

CHAPTER TEN

Marathon Man

*T*wo months after I started my cleanse, in January 2010, Melissa thought we should add some cardiovascular work to my strength training. She suggested I start doing some light running. I suggested she jump up my . . .

I am not a runner. Don't wanna be a runner. Could care less about running. It's always been a source of contention between me and Deborah. And sometimes, I would feel guilty when she would come downstairs on a Saturday morning, looking hot in her running togs and me sitting in the kitchen in my pj's. But that would pass about ten seconds after she left to go be healthy.

Now here's Melissa suggesting I start . . . running.

So I did.

Why?

Because it seemed like the easiest way for me to get my much-needed cardio training in. I didn't like it. But I had to do it. I am

••

also not crazy about having to watch what I eat, but again, I have to do it. These two things seem to go hand in hand.

I started with a mile at first. It took twenty minutes. Whooooeeee. Did you hear that sonic boom? It was a little disheartening in the beginning, but I kept at it. After a couple of weeks I got that mile down to nineteen minutes, then eighteen. After two months, and regular mileage goals determined by Melissa, I was doing a fourteen-minute mile. Not world-class, but better than I was.

As I have mentioned, I am a gadget guy. I love technology. I am what they call an early adopter. I had a Pulsar watch, a Casio BOSS, a Sony digital camera with a floppy disk, and an Apple Newton. Knowing this, Melissa suggested I get a running watch. I did my research and I got a Garmin 405 training watch.

While Deborah can throw on a pair of sneakers and just go for a run, I can't. I need a regimen—a set routine and someone to push me to the limit. The watch helped me by tracking my training and then sending the information to my computer and to Melissa, who would monitor and adjust my workouts based on the data. It continuously monitors your time, distance, pace, calories and even your heart rate when paired with a heart rate monitor. Each run is stored in memory so you can review and analyze the data to see how you've improved. You can even download recorded courses to compete against previous workouts.

Then in a late February phone call, Melissa floated an idea that would change my life.

"You know," she said, "the way you're running, you could do a marathon."

"Excuse me?" I replied. "There's something wrong. You're breaking up. It sounded like you said I could run a marathon!"

She was laughing as she answered, "You can do this. Your times are good; your endurance is getting better. You CAN run a marathon."

I know what you're thinking.

Al Roker . . . the guy who hates to work out, who believes doing *nothing* is best, who never ran by choice—*that* Al Roker running a marathon?

Yup.

I never considered myself to be an "athlete." I only started jogging as part of my nutritional program with Melissa, to get a little cardio into my routine. Perhaps the cleanse had made my thinking a little too clear! Suddenly, I was thinking of things that were way out of my comfort zone.

Or was it?

I'm a somewhat competitive guy, and since losing the weight, I was looking for something new to challenge myself.

Hmm. If I agreed, I knew I'd have to get Deborah on board with the idea, too. You see, Deborah is the runner in our family. She has been a runner all of her life. She's that athlete who gets a thrill from training. Me? Not so much.

Melissa suggested a compromise. "The Rock 'n' Roll Half Marathon in Chicago is coming up in August. We'll train for that and see how you do. Then we can reevaluate for the New York City Marathon."

I was working with a crazy woman. She was actually suggesting, out loud, that I run the New York City Marathon?

So I answered with the only thing I could say.

"Yes."

When I told Deborah I was thinking about doing the Chicago half–marathon to test the waters, she was supportive but skeptical. And with good reason. You see, I have really bad knees as a result of a horrific car accident in 1985. I was driving home on the Saw Mill River Parkway when a woman made a left turn into the oncoming traffic. I slammed into her head-on. My upper leg drove down into my lower leg, shattering my knee and tibia. I was wearing my favorite Oxford chalk stripe suit I'd bought at Wallach's. When the paramedics told me they had to cut the pant leg off to get to my injuries, I screamed, "NO!!" as loud as I could. They thought I was in pain, but I was really upset about losing the suit. Why hadn't I worn a blue blazer and khaki pants that day?

After I was stabilized at Westchester Medical Center, we consulted with a number of doctors in Westchester and New York City, and the consensus was that I might have to lose my leg or at best I would need a brace and walk with a cane for the rest of my life.

A family friend suggested we see a brilliant young orthopedic surgeon at Phelps Memorial Hospital in Westchester. Dr. Bob Seebacher was cocky and brash, and he saved my leg. We remain good friends to this day. He and his team were able to rebuild my leg using clamps and screws. Afterward, Bob told me I would have an arthritic knee that would likely require knee replacement surgery in five or six years. (He was right. While I held off for as long as I could, I eventually had a knee replacement in March 2001—sixteen years after the accident.)

I should have been in the hospital for two months, but I was released after just a few weeks and was back to work a month later. I even lost a little weight. It wasn't especially hard—my extended hospital stay made it challenging for me to eat the way I normally did. And besides, anyone who has ever been in the hospital knows the food is pretty awful.

Anyway, knowing my history, Deborah was legitimately worried that a marathon—even a half marathon—might be too much stress on my knees. She offered her total support as long as I could get the approval of Dr. Riley Williams, a good friend of ours who is an orthopedic surgeon as well as the team doctor for the New Jersey Nets and Devils. She was pretty sure he'd never sign off!

We first met Riley when Leila suffered a knee injury from playing kickball. He has the absolute best bedside manner with kids I have ever seen. But he can also be a real guy's guy. Imagine Chris Rock as your surgeon—with no censor. That's how Riley can be with patients like me.

When I went to see him to discuss my marathon training, he started right in, very mellow.

"So, your old lady calls me and she wants me to talk you out of doing the marathon. Here's how I feel—you want to run this motherfucker, then run this motherfucker. I will get you through this motherfucker. If you tell me you want to do this mother-fucking training every other weekend, I am going to tell you that you are out of your motherfucking mind. But if you want to run it, I say run it."

So, you know what I did?

I decided to run that motherfucker!

But first, I would have to train. Riley prescribed an anti-inflammatory to take after running and made me promise to stretch and ice my knees every day.

By this time, I had gotten my average mile down to around thirteen minutes. I will never forget my very first really long run, which was six miles. It was late March and our family was in the Bahamas for spring break. The temperature was unbearably hot, around 92 degrees, and so humid I could barely breathe. I kept thinking to myself, "What am I doing?" Still, I had to run the miles as part of my training or I'd fall behind. I was sweating like crazy. But when I finished, I felt a great sense of accomplishment—and I gratefully took a plunge in the pool to cool off!

I really don't enjoy running in heat—my ideal weather for running is about 55 degrees, sunny and no wind!—but I found myself doing it a lot because I had to train all that summer. The worst experience I had running in high temperatures was during a visit to see Deborah's family in Perry, Georgia. It was 96 degrees out with 60 percent humidity. The air was thick and still. I had to run sixteen miles that day. I drove the course I planned to run and planted bottles of water every two miles along the way so I could keep myself hydrated. I would never have made the entire run if I didn't do that in advance.

I took off early that Saturday morning, before the heat became unbearable. I didn't see another runner the entire time. Whenever I stopped for water, someone would pull over and ask me if I was okay.

"Y'all okay?"

"Yes, fine. Thanks!"

"Everything all right?"

"Yup. Good. Thanks."

Somewhere around the fifteen-mile marker, I was wiped out, so I stopped to catch my breath. When you run long distances or do a strenuous extended workout, your body loses essential vitamins and minerals. One of those is potassium. Potassium works with sodium to maintain the body's water balance. A normal level of potassium in the blood is important so that your cells, nerves, heart, muscles, and kidneys work properly. I always kept potassium tablets with me when I ran and take them as needed—and in that moment, I definitely needed it. I was also sucking back these foil packets of nutrition called Gu. So I looked great . . . chugging water, swallowing pills and sucking on a foil packet. Drinker? Druggie? Whatever!

So I was standing there on the side of the road, hunched over with my hands on my knees, when an old man pulled over in his pickup truck.

"You okay?" he asked.

"Yes, I'm fine," I panted. Then a state trooper pulled over. I couldn't imagine what he wanted. I was just a guy out for a run!

"Sir, you look a little pale." Now, coming from a cop, in the South, I wasn't really sure how to take that. I wasn't looking for any trouble, so I assured him I was fine and headed back to the hotel. When I got there, I looked in the mirror and to my shock my face looked, well, *white!* I had been sweating so much that the sweat evaporated and left a layer of salt all over my face. The trooper was right! I did look pale!

By the time August came around, I was ready for the half-marathon. To keep me motivated, Melissa and her marathon running partner, Jared Svoboda, ran the entire course with me, which I completed in 3:20. I took Deborah and the kids along and made a weekend out of it, which made it fun for all of us. My buddy Jon Harris came out with his family as well. I love Jon. He is my brother from another mother. We both love life, our families and good music. (And we're both married to health freaks who have less than 3 percent body fat. Jon's wife, Allie, runs ten miles a day.)

When I finished the half-marathon, Melissa said she thought I could actually run and finish the New York City Marathon—the largest marathon in the world.

"Are you nuts?" I asked.

Apparently not. But obviously, I am.

••

Melissa explained that my numbers were all on track to do it. The race takes place on the first Sunday of November, so I still had two and a half months to train for it. If it became too much, I promised everyone I would stop. Even though she was getting over a hamstring injury, Meredith Vieira, who was also working with Melissa, agreed to get on board and run the marathon with me. It would be nice to have a familiar face to run with on the big day, even though, given the difference between Meredith's speed and mine, I would see her face at the beginning of the race, then her butt and then she'd be gone.

Training for a full 26.2-mile marathon is a commitment of colossal proportions. But being the slightly obsessive guy that I am, once I get on a routine, I am in it to win it. And when I say "win" I mean finish: making it to the finish line without either throwing up or pooping my shorts, as some world-class athletes have actually done. That is a "win" to me.

If you decide to train for something like a marathon, it's important that you have a great support system of people who understand the amount of time it takes to prepare. The one thing we all have that is finite is our time, so the time you devote to training and working out is time taken away from other things, including your family. If you don't have a supportive spouse or family, it can be very difficult to choose between your training and them. As you go into this kind of endeavor, you need to talk to your significant other and explain what this means to you. Let them know your training has nothing to do with wanting to be away from the family; it's about doing something healthy and good for you. It's not selfish, so don't get caught up feeling guilty, or you will never get past it and succeed.

In the old days, if something came up in my schedule, my workouts were the first thing I'd cancel. These days, I know I need to put myself first if I'm going to stay on my path. Look, if all else fails, try making the family a part of your training as a way to include them in the process. There were plenty of times I'd do a short run with my son before heading out for a longer, more grueling one. Even if you have to do a walk/run to get some time together, in the end, it's all worth it.

Once I committed to the idea of doing a full marathon, I slowly began adding mileage to my training, going from six-mile runs up to twelve, thirteen and sixteen miles, which could sometimes take me five or six hours to complete. Even though it meant taking an entire Saturday away from my wife and kids, there was no way Deborah could be upset with me for training for a marathon! After all, she had loved the idea of my taking up running. Of course, the occasional jog turned into two miles a couple of days a week, turned into ten miles on a weekday and eventually fifteen- or twenty-mile runs on weekends. I'd read an article in the *Wall Street Journal* about workout widows—women whose relationships suffer because of their husbands' exercise. But Deborah was my rock. She always supported me and believed in my commitment to our relationship.

I saved my long runs for weekends at our home in upstate New York. Just as I had done in Georgia, I'd plot out my course every weekend by driving our family minivan. The night before, I placed bottles of water every two miles along the planned route. (When I finished my run, I'd drive back and pick up all of my empty bottles!) One weekend, someone actually stole two bottles of my water along the way. I had to run into the local deli to buy water. It's a good thing I always carry a little cash with me!

Since my wife is a runner, one might think we spent hours training together—but we didn't. We have never trained well together because she loves to work out and I pretty much loathe it. Whenever we'd go for a run together, we always ended up in a fight or some kind of disagreement. In short distances, Deborah could easily outrun me. She is a better runner than I am and much faster; but of course I was training for distance, not speed.

In September, Deborah and I had planned a long weekend in Paris together to celebrate our fifteenth anniversary. It happened to coincide with an eighteen-mile run I needed to squeeze in for my training. I Googled the perfect scenic course around the city, including a run along the Seine. When Deborah woke up, she said she wanted to run with me.

Uh-oh.

I love my wife dearly, but every bit of me knew it wouldn't end well because the longest she had run was six miles or so. I just couldn't say no, so she got dressed and we headed out.

"Let's get going," Deborah said, jogging in place, raring to go.

But I wasn't ready yet. My Garmin 410 (I had moved up to a new model) hadn't picked up the GPS satellite signal yet, something that was important to me to do the run as planned. Deborah started complaining. "Let's go. Don't worry about your watch." But I know me. I could not really do my best unless that watch was running. It finally kicked in and we were off.

It was beautiful. It was a crisp, clear morning as we ran the streets of Paris along the path next to the Seine. We jogged past Nôtre Dame, across a bridge over the river and eventually past the Eiffel Tower.

At around mile six, I asked Deborah how long she planned to run with me.

"You don't think I can do it, do you?" she said, and picked up her pace.

It wasn't that I didn't think she could keep up. I was worried she would overdo it. I had been training for months. I was used to running on all types of surfaces, but Paris is a city full of cobblestone streets, which can be very harsh on the ankles, shins and knees.

At mile seven, I asked her again, "How long until you peel off?"

Deborah is far more competitive than I am. "Just because you *think* you're a runner," she said. "I'll show you I can run!"

It was interesting that Deborah said I *thought* of myself as a runner because I was such a slug for so many years. We would go on vacations and she would bring her workout gear and I wouldn't even bring sneakers. Now here we were in Paris for a romantic weekend, and I had all of my gear to train for a marathon.

It wasn't until mile eight that she finally gave up. I love her for wanting to stay with me that day, but in the end, it took her knees almost a year to recover from banging over those cobblestones, which annoyed her even more. The very idea that I ran eighteen miles and she was a hurtin' buckaroo after eight just pissed her off to a fare-thee-well.

I have learned a lot over the course of my three marriages, and one of the greatest lessons I've learned is there is no satisfaction in "I told you so's!" Pick your battles or you will inevitably lose the war. It's a good thing we have such a solid relationship because training as hard as you do for a marathon can put a lot of stress on even the best marriage. Like I said earlier, happy wife, happy life. Thankfully, Deborah never made me choose between doing something that made her happy over making myself happy. Now, *that's* unconditional love and support.

I will be completely honest and tell you that I pretty much hated the entire training process. I'd heard people talk about this thing called the "runner's high" but I never got that—never.

Meredith always teased me about that. She was a serious runner and we became kindred spirits who would come to the studio on Monday mornings to compare notes on our runs. The emotional support was a tremendous help, and from my perspective created a really special bond.

Sunday morning, November 6, 2010, dawned clear, cool and almost cloudless (said the weatherman!). Meredith and I and our team of Melissa Bowman Li and Jared Svoboda rode over together to the Staten Island side of the Verrazano-Narrows Bridge at Fort Wadsworth Park, the staging area for the forty thousand runners and the starting point for the race. The plan was for Melissa to run with Meredith and Jared to run with me. He is a world-class marathoner. Two weeks earlier, he had run two marathons in two days to raise money for the Make-A-Wish Foundation. He was loose and cool as a cucumber. I, on the other hand, was uptight and nervous. Before the race, people were coming up to me asking, "What time are you looking to do?"

Time? Are you crazy? I just wanted to finish the darn thing!

Another guy said to me before the race, "Don't burn yourself out on First Avenue, because you're going to really want to start running to the finish line."

I shook my head thinking, "Not running so much as crawling."

I didn't have a clue what I had signed up for. I looked at the Verrazano-Narrows Bridge and wondered, "What was I thinking?"

But there was no backing out so I got myself into the "Let's go!" mind-set before I could possibly change my mind.

I knew Deborah, Leila, Nicky, Courtney, my brother Chris, his wife, Latice, and my nephew André would be there along First Avenue to cheer me on. I was ready, determined and prepared to do this thing! When the corral started off and I began running, my adrenaline kicked right in and got me going. I was literally off to the races. It wasn't until I got to Brooklyn that I realized just how many hills there are in and around New York. That said, it was a thrilling experience. You get to see the five boroughs of New York City up close and personal, with total strangers urging you on. I wanted to make sure I drank it all in, stopping along the way to take pictures with people and of places.

One of the hardest sections was the Queensboro Bridge, where you run on the lower level and it's a mostly uphill climb. There's almost nobody cheering you on. Then suddenly there's a drop, bales of hay and a sharp turn onto First Avenue. Hay bales?? Like they're expecting Indy 500–like crashes.

Running up First Avenue was tough, although seeing my family cheering along the side of the road meant the world to me. It gave me that incentive to go on despite the fact that I was cramping up a bit and was worried I wouldn't have the stamina to finish the race. Running with a non–New Yorker like Jared helped pass the time with my pointing out various landmarks and points of interest along the way. Poor Melissa running with Meredith—a woman who has been in NYC for something like thirty years and knows nothing about the town. Meredith was telling Melissa about Queens when they were in the Bronx. Sheesh!

Although Meredith and I started the race together, after the first fifteen minutes, she took off ahead of me and I never saw her again along the course until the finish line, an hour and ten minutes after she crossed it.

As the sun was setting and the course started to darken, I turned off Central Park South and back into Central Park toward the finish line. As I approached it, I could see my family and friends. There was Nicky running up to greet me, then Deborah, Courtney and Leila. I saw Chris and Latice with André, and my friend Stephanie Abrams, my cohost on the Weather Channel, who had also shown up to support me. And there, waiting for me, were my running partners Meredith and Melissa. We group-hugged and kissed and I started crying. I thought about my mother and my father. How proud they would have been to witness this feat. I mean, deep down, I know they saw it from where they are, but I missed having them there. And at that moment, I knew that I had kept my promise to my father.

My final time was 7:09:44. Not a world-beater. In fact, Leila said, "Dad, it's kind of like what the snail said on top of the turtle." I'll bite. "What was that, sweetheart?" I asked. "Wheeeeeeeeee!" she said, laughing.

Since the marathon, I've kept up with my running. I try to get two runs in during the week after the *Today* show and two longer runs early in the morning on weekends. When I'm in New York, I enjoy running along the Hudson River up to the George Washington Bridge and back down to Battery Park. I generally run by myself, although I am never really alone because I listen to my iPod, which has every type of music on it from Stevie Wonder to Billy Joel to the Black Eyed Peas and Elton John. I've got some Pink, Beyoncé, Nicki Minaj, Cee Lo Green, Lady Gaga, Usher and Flo Rida on there, too! Running is now a favorite time, when I can quietly mull over a problem or just let my mind go blank and take in the scenery of wherever I am. Not long ago, I took a quick trip to Australia to do a story for the *Today* show and had the chance to run along the harbor in the warm Aussie breeze. It was glorious!

Occasionally, my runs have taken me on some unexpected adventures, too! While running in Greenough, Montana, I came across a bear cub. I thought to myself, "If there's a bear cub, there's a mother bear somewhere nearby!" I knew if I kept going that park rangers would eventually come across my sneakers and that's about all they'd find, so I doubled back to the lodge where I was staying, arriving in one piece!

While writing this book, I decided to take on yet another physical challenge I never thought I'd do: train for a triathlon. I've now incorporated swimming into my running and biking and plan to participate in a mini-triathlon in the fall of 2012. But my knees have been acting up lately, which means I will probably have to pay a visit to Dr. Riley. Motherfucker!

In the meantime, I've been keeping up with my biking. In fact, when I went to London to cover the 2012 Summer Olympic games, I brought along my portable Brompton bike, which folds up to the size of a large briefcase. The bike is actually made in England, where they are quite common. I brought it with me as a way to avoid the anticipated traffic and keep up my physical fitness without putting too much pressure on my knees. It's very light and easy to take on the subway or bus or put in the trunk of a cab. It was kind of cute bringing my bike home to see where it was born, and there's not a better way to see London or any city than from the vantage point on two wheels.

CHAPTER ELEVEN

Saboteurs

*T*here are things in life that have the potential to ruin your dieting resolve every time; I believe that forewarned is forearmed. Saboteurs come in many shapes, sizes and forms and they're always present when you are trying to make a life-altering change. It was absolutely devastating to read the hospital description of me as "morbidly obese"—far worse than someone calling me a fatso or lard ass—but even now that I've lost weight I'm still being criticized. Every now and then people in the Twittersphere will post something along the lines of "I liked Al Roker better when he was fat." Or "I liked the old Al Roker better."

Really?

Did you wake up this morning with a sudden epiphany that a fat weatherman is smarter, funnier, more likable—or just more like you?

What exactly was better about me weighing three hundred forty pounds?

Did my weight somehow make you feel better about your own appearance?

There was a time in my life where these types of comments could have derailed me—triggering an eating binge of colossal proportions! That may have been true in the past, but not anymore. Sometimes I'll tweet back a quick response saying, "That guy is never coming back—get used to it" or "Too bad, because I'm never going back to being fat." I don't think it means much to them, but it helps me to feel strong and secure that I'm in a great place in my life and that what other people think doesn't really matter. I'm hardly the only person I know who's been hurt by a casual comment. I grew up in a culture where women had sexy curves and there was a social acceptance of that body type. My grandmother told my ex-wife that she liked her better with a little meat on her bones. While my grandmother meant it as a compliment, my ex-wife took offense because she felt she was being called fat.

Before my surgery, people felt free to heckle me all the time for being fat. Others used to stop me on the street to say, "You look so much better in person," and think it was a compliment— but it's not. What they're really saying is that on TV I'm frightening but in person, I'm not so bad! Okay, I know they didn't mean it the way it sounds but it didn't sting any less. That's why I usually find it's better to say nothing more than a "hello" or "nice to see you" when I bump into people I haven't seen for a while. This way, I don't risk saying something well intended but actually offensive.

It's common for folks to regard TV personalities as relatable: more "everyday people" than, say, movie stars. It's an intimate relationship in a funny way. So a lot of people feel as though they can blurt out things to me they'd never say to a stranger, like they'll see me walking down the street eating an apple and shout, "Hey, you sure you want to eat that?"

Most probably meant well, but to be honest, they could afford to push away from the table, too! And others who didn't mean so well may have wanted to feel a false sense of physical and mental superiority, like they have more self-control than I do. Maybe they thought, "Look at this fat guy on TV—I could do what he does!"

Wittingly or unwittingly, people are going to make comments; it's your choice how to react. Trust me; they will go on with their day without a care in the world.

But will you?

Whether it's a conscious attempt to derail your progress or not, you are in control of the aftermath. Is undoing everything you have worked so hard to achieve worth a binge? If you still aren't sure, try measuring your success against their comment. Don't let a fleeting moment wreck weeks, months or even years of progress.

You can even sabotage yourself out of concern for someone else. When you're in a relationship with someone who lives the same sedentary lifestyle you do, it might feel like an insult or a rejection to try to lose weight and get in shape. Lucky for me, I'm married to a woman who values a healthy lifestyle and goes out of her way to support me and our kids in pursuit of that goal. I once heard a story about a woman who lost over one hundred pounds and her husband felt so insecure about her new size that he bought her candy and a size XXXX shirt for Christmas.

People become saboteurs for many different reasons. For some, it's about control, or the fear of losing control. Others simply feel threatened. *You* on a diet makes *them* feel bad about their own weight. If you're ready to change and they're not, they may do whatever they can to talk you out of it, because of their own fears. It's like a lobster pot—if one lobster tries to crawl out of the boiling water, the others will pull him back in so they all die together.

Then there are those friends who are just plain old competitive. If you're succeeding at something, even if it's losing weight, they feel it makes them look less successful. And when it comes to the office, they might even fear you're going to beat them out for a promotion because surely your boss will take notice that you've gained control over your health. I remember one night inviting a friend over who knew I was trying to lose weight. We were in the kitchen preparing dinner together when she started putting avocado in my salad. While I don't think her intentions were bad, I got angry because avocado has a lot of fat in it. Granted, it's the good type of fat, but I didn't want *any* fats! To her, it was just a few slices of avocado, but to me it was an attempt to sabotage my progress.

When you make a drastic change in your lifestyle, there is always going to be someone who isn't comfortable with the new you. They've gotten used to you as a bigger person; they've grown accustomed to the way you look. When you change that up for yourself, you are also changing it up for them and that can be hard.

When I worked at WNBC, we had a stage manager who always dressed like a schlep and had a long scraggly beard that made him look like an unkempt rabbi. One day, the producer decided to give him a makeover for a segment. They cut his hair, took out the gray, put him in some nice clothes and made him unrecognizably handsome. Everyone at the studio thought he looked amazing. And he really did.

The guy loved his new look and couldn't wait to go home and show his wife. He was about to take a month off for his annual vacation, and left feeling like a million bucks. When he came back to work thirty days later, he had reverted back to the old him. His wife had hated the new look because she worried others might find him attractive and he would leave her. Happy wife, happy life—so he went back to his old look. I think this happens a lot. When people feel threatened, they fight back. Some people are equipped for the battle, but most of the time, they never even saw it coming.

While people are the most obvious saboteurs of dieting, plain old life can get in the way of your success, too. A lot of people use the holidays as an excuse to let go and let live. I used to be one of those guys. I was always pretty good about Thanksgiving, because it's a one-day holiday, but December always seemed to bring a plethora of parties and pastries to tempt even the strongest willed. Even now, my weight can fluctuate twenty pounds around the holidays if I am not cautious and conscious of my eating.

Eating out can also make it harder to stay the course. We've long known that restaurant meals aren't a paragon of healthy portion sizes, but a new study shows they may be even worse than we think. According to a study published in the journal *Public Health Nutrition*, a whopping 96 percent of America's chain restaurant entrées fall outside the range of the USDA's recommendations for fat, saturated fat and sodium per meal. When you eat out, your chances of finding an entrée that's truly healthy are painfully low.

The RAND Corporation "evaluated 28,433 regular menu items and 1,833 children's menus at 245 restaurants around the country between February and May 2010," and discovered that "while the majority of dishes fell below the USDA's calorie limit for a meal (667 calories), they did not meet the requirements for fat, saturated fat and sodium (which, according to the government regulations, should not exceed 767 mg per meal). Many items may appear healthy based on calories, but can be very unhealthy when you consider other important nutrition criteria." According to the study, "sodium, in particular, was problematic . . . [with] the average dinner entrée [packing] a whopping 1,512 mg, more than the CDC's recommended adequate intake . . . (and not too far from their recommended *maximum* intake of 2,300 mg)." Fast-food restaurants usually get the brunt of this type of research, but the truth is most family style restaurants are major culprits, too, according to the report, which went on to say:

"And don't think you're doing your diet any favors by ordering an appetizer instead of a main dish; the researchers reported that those meal 'starters' often had more calories, fat and sodium than any other item on the menu."

Restaurants use butter and oil on almost everything because aside from making your food taste better, it makes it look more appetizing, too. If you're trying to lose weight, adjust your schedule to eat at home more frequently than eating out. And if you have to eat out, make sure you ask for your food to be prepared without butter or oil, including your salads. A common dieting mistake is ordering a healthy salad and then slathering it with fattening dressing.

A lack of sleep can also throw off even the best-laid plan.

When you are sleep deprived, you tend to eat more, make poorer food choices and exercise less. Boy, I'm in the perfect job, huh? Go to bed at ten p.m. and get up at three-fifteen each morning. Pass me those Lorna Doones, will ya?

Being tired and less active was definitely one of my triggers to make the wrong choices. It takes less energy to order in Chinese food than it is to cook up a broiled chicken breast and steam some broccoli. But easy and convenient aren't always your friends when it comes to losing weight—especially when you're tired.

I don't enjoy exercising on a good day, but when I am exhausted, it's the last thing I feel like doing. If I give in to my fatigue, I will pay the price by not burning extra calories that day. Plus, a recent study published in *International Journal of Workplace Health Management* states that "people who exercised are more productive and in a better mood, especially at work, than those who didn't exercise." It's important to remember that exercise keeps the mind sharp and your spirits up, and that's a benefit to everyone.

Anyone who has ever been on a diet knows that boredom is the breeding ground for bad habits. When I was working at WNBC, there were many nights on the drive home after the eleven o'clock news that I'd slam down a dozen Krispy Kreme donuts, or a couple of Quarter Pounders, two large orders of fries and a vanilla shake. I might have been a little hungry, but mostly this was a habit I developed to fulfill me on the drive home. There were no cell phones back then, so I ate instead of talking to someone to pass the time. I certainly didn't need to eat all of that food, but it gave me something to do. About ten minutes before I got home, I would roll the car windows down so I didn't smell like McDonald's (we all know that smell!) and I always threw the wrappers away before walking through the front door. I didn't want my wife to know I was sucking down three thousand calories every night after work.

This was typical of my eating habits. If the only calories I took in came from the food I ate in public, I would have been fit and trim. My problem was never what I was eating in front of others; it was the amount of food I was consuming when no one else was around. Oh yeah. I was a big-time closet eater. True closet eaters are usually severely overweight. Shame, guilt, and severe depression are common after a binge, especially if you're trying to lose weight. Plus, it sets up an unhealthy cycle. After a bout of closet eating, the negative emotions that triggered the binge in the first place return along with guilt about the setback to weight loss. This can lead to more depression, resulting in more closet eating. My emotional binges became a big part of the vicious cycle I found myself in every time I went on any type of diet. I'd lose weight, gain it back and get so mad at myself for failing that I'd eat something to make myself feel better. As soon as that food was gone, I felt so bad that I beat myself up for being so stupid and self-destructive. The worse I made myself feel, the more I'd turn to food for comfort. It was a never-ending circle that kept leading me back to where I started—fat and miserable.

In a way, I equate the shame and guilt associated with closet eating to being an alcoholic who has a couple of drinks in the bar before going home and then tries to hide the smell of booze on his breath, or a closet smoker who pretends you can't smell the smoke on his clothes. For me, that meant rolling down the windows in the dead of winter so my wife couldn't smell McDonald's in the car or on me. Let me tell you, that was a pretty cold breeze late at night in subzero temperatures just to hide that I had just eaten a couple of burgers.

Health professionals have only recently recognized closet eating as a disorder and as a subset of binge eating, which is a newly recognized eating disorder itself. Binging is defined as eating larger than normal amounts of food, usually with a feeling of loss of control over eating, and without throwing up afterward. The same holds true for closet eating, but closet eaters only binge when they're alone because they feel ashamed or embarrassed to overeat in front of other people. No one is really sure what causes closet eating, but many experts believe it may be due to bad memories related to eating and weight, especially if you were ridiculed about your body or reprimanded for eating too much as a child. The result is shame about eating in public, which triggers the excessive eating as a way to find comfort or drown the negative emotions.

By now you know the stories of burgers in the car, but my secret eating went way beyond driving. Whenever I'd go on the road for work, I'd find myself in nice hotels all over the world, with great restaurants—and room service. So I could order fine cuisine and enjoy it in the comfort and privacy of my room with no one to watch what I was eating. I wasn't overeating so much as overindulging. I'd order creamy, gooey, sauce-laden dishes I'd never order in front of my wife because I wanted her to believe that I was trying to be good.

Road trips are always fun, but when it comes to dieting, they were a real stumbling block for me. Traveling for the *Today* show, we'd often eat breakfast together at the hotel or on the set, where there was usually a cooking segment involved. I'd throw back a stack of pancakes and a slab of bacon every morning, then eat again on the set. For dinner, we'd usually end up in a steak house or some other fine restaurant where in the celebratory spirit I'd throw caution to the wind, ordering a New York strip and creamed spinach without giving any thought to the amount of calories I was consuming.

Being on the road can be especially bad when you're not doing your regular (or any) exercise, and at the time, I was as sedentary as I was fat. A couple of days eating with wild abandon will quickly take its toll. While I will admit that I am an emotional eater, at the end of the day, I am also just a guy who *really likes food*. I like cooking it, eating it, reading about it and shopping for it.

One of the greatest benefits of being on the *Today* show is meeting the world-class chefs who come through our studio kitchen. Watching them elevates my interest in cuisine even more. Unfortunately, many mornings, as soon as our segment with a well-known chef had ended, I'd find myself hiding in my dressing room chowing down on a full plate full of yumminess I didn't want anyone to see me eating. I remember when the great Cajun chef Paul Prudhomme came on the show once I thought, "Geez, I hope I never get as big as this guy!" He was a little shorter than I was and, from my perspective, appeared to be much bigger than me. In retrospect, I have to admit, we could have been the same size and I would have never known it.

It took me many years to fully understand that my overeating was a by-product of all of these factors. But while there are plenty of *outside* sources for sabotaging your path to health and fitness, usually the biggest and most challenging hurdle we have to get past is *ourselves*.

BINGE/CLOSET EATING

THE EXACT NUMBER OF PEOPLE WHO HAVE THIS DISORDER is unknown, but a recent study reported that eating disorders other than anorexia, along with abnormal attitudes about food, affect 10 to 15 percent of women. In that study of 1,500 women, 13.7 percent admitted to binging one to seven times per month. About 75 percent of eating disorders are caused by emotions. Additionally, an underlying psychological disorder, such as depression, may be contributing to the closet eating.

This type of emotional eating is easy to recognize. Besides a preference for eating alone, other common symptoms of closet eating are:

➤ Feeling shame and embarrassment about eating in public

➤ Binging on comfort foods, junk foods and sweets when alone

➤ Hoarding food and hiding empty food containers

➤ Eating a large amount of food in one sitting

➤ Feeling powerless to stop eating

➤ Binging but not purging

CHAPTER TWELVE

The Best Advice Is No Advice

As long as there is food, there will always be diets. I've spent most of my life proving that diets simply don't work. I've been on every fad diet known to man and spent thousands of dollars in the hope that those diets would somehow be my magic bullet, but instead destined me for failure. The inevitable return of the pounds I lost, and often additional pounds, made me think permanent weight loss was very difficult to achieve if not completely impossible.

That's why I've become a former dieter.

What's the point?

By now you know that this isn't a book about weight loss so much as it is my story of how I finally discovered my path to good health and fitness. You won't find a lot of diet "advice" in these pages—just my own experiences that led me to where I am today. I understand how fat people think because I've been on every side of the diet cycle. I've been the fat guy who envies the thin guys, and the fat guy who says take me as I am. I've been the thin guy who swore I'd never gain back the weight. I've been the jealous guy who thought someone else losing weight meant I was a failure. I've secretly rooted for the newly skinny dude to gain it all back because I was struggling and he was doing well and then reveled in my satisfaction when he put his weight back on. Gosh, that kind of makes me sound like a jerk, doesn't it? Yet many of you reading this are probably nodding your heads in agreement because you have been in these same situations. If you're going to get anything from this book, I'm hoping you will embrace my honesty and find some solace that you are not alone on this journey. I have chosen not to hold back because it's a road we've all traveled, and you can't know where you're going if you don't know where you've been.

Although I've been fairly public about my struggles with weight over the years, I've made it a point to avoid offering diet advice to anyone. My sister recently asked me to talk to my baby brother about losing weight because she thought he might listen to me. After all, been there, done that, right? Well, here's the thing. I am the last person he wants to hear it from. I wouldn't do it even if I hadn't lost weight. Most people think that talking to someone about losing weight motivates that person, but it does just the opposite. If merely "bringing up" the topic worked, I would have lost weight a long time ago!

Here's the only real advice I am going to offer all of you out there who are reading this book with the hope that you will get a loved one to lose weight:

SHUT YOUR MOUTH!

They know they are fat.

You hammering them makes that person feel worse about themselves and usually leads to eating more.

People who don't struggle with their weight don't have a clue what it's like to go through life thinking about our girth every waking moment, yet they feel the need to lecture, judge and offer unsolicited opinions we don't want to hear. It's like a sober guy trying to convince a drunk not to drink. It doesn't work. If it did, AA wouldn't exist.

Even though my wife, Deborah, has never struggled with her weight, I remember when she was pregnant with our daughter Leila. I told her that there would be people in her life who secretly hoped she would have a little trouble dropping the baby weight after giving birth. Most of those people would be friends or family members who struggle with their own weight, who unconsciously or not were just waiting for Deborah to have to get a little taste of what they struggle with every day. Deborah thought I was nuts. She didn't think it was possible for anyone to wish that on her—but I knew it was, because I'd seen it happen so many times in my life. Thankfully, she was in such terrific shape when she got pregnant that it was relatively easy for her to get her old body back. But just as I had predicted, she began to hear comments like "I can't believe you didn't struggle" and "I thought for sure you'd have problems taking off the baby weight!" Deborah admitted she was absolutely shocked that I was right; obviously, she'd forgotten that I was the Mayor of Fat City for several successive terms. Thankfully, term limits kicked in!

It's critical to your success to understand that no one is responsible for making you feel good about yourself except YOU. Deborah and I have had many discussions about the role of a spouse or partner when it comes to weight loss. This battle has been known to sink a marriage or two. For most couples, weight loss is a game changer because it disrupts the designated roles in the relationship. But even when the thin partner genuinely wants to help, it's often ineffective and frustrating. All that concern about the fat partner's weight, the urging him to eat right and exercise more, show a little more willpower, try a little harder, the assurance that if only he could get thin then everything would be all right . . . it's not good for the relationship.

Why?

Because 95 percent of people who go on diets fail.

Maybe they should start an Occupy Dunkin Donuts movement against the 5 percent who succeed!

A marriage is tested by many things. One person's weight is not the be all and end all. My wife is ecstatic with how I look these days but it wasn't an easy road for either of us to get here. I always tell my single friends that they are better off with someone like me than with the hunky Matt Lauer type because eventually they are going to lose their looks, maybe even gain weight. (Except for Matt. He will always look as good as he does. I hate him.) (No. Not really.) (Well, not much.) Anyway, with guys like me, there's a baseline, a certain understanding going in that this is as bad as it gets. See, we have nowhere to go but up. We start working out, lose some pounds . . . and you end up with a new man!

Deborah knew who I was when she married me. I have joked that I knew she was really in love with me because she let me get on top of her—even at my worst. But once I lost the weight for good, our relationship got even better than we could ever have imagined when we got married. For me, I no longer had to beg my wife for sex and for the first time in years, I could look down and see my—feet. The better I looked, the more turned on she got and the better shot I had at getting some. What great motivation to keep looking good. It was like Pavlov's dog, and kind of a no-brainer.

All kidding aside, fat people who get thin are reborn. They want all of the benefits and acceptance that being thin grants and they never want to be the fat man in the room again. To be successful, they know they can never go back to their old ways and habits without regaining the weight, which means leaving the past behind. If the other person in the relationship can't accept that, it may not end the way you hoped. The decision to finally get a hold on your health and wellness is one of the most important you'll ever make in your life—but it takes commitment, willpower and a willingness to sacrifice a lot of things you've gotten used to for many years.

It took Deborah many years to understand that my battle of the bulge is not her fight. Learning to say nothing was one of the hardest realizations she had to come to. Thankfully, she embraced the new me and became my biggest supporter and cheerleader to stay on my newfound path after losing the weight—but when I started to gain some of that weight back, when I reverted to my old habits, hers came back, too. This became a lesson in patience and acceptance for both of us. For me, it was about once again gaining control over my eating, and for Deborah, it was about letting go. Letting me make the decision to get back in the saddle.

To help you better understand what it's like for the other person in your life to be along for the ride, I asked Deborah to share some of her "do's" and "don'ts" that have helped us in our relationship and created a much happier space at home together.

Deborah's Do's and Don'ts for a Happier Home

➤ Don't assume the fight is yours, because it's not.

➤ Don't judge your spouse for what he's eating even when you know it is the wrong thing. He knows it's wrong. I tried being the food police for years, and it was awful. Nobody likes to be policed, especially a grown man. If you can remove yourself from the struggle, there will be more harmony in your home and in your relationship. The other person might even feel freer to eventually make the right decision.

➤ Do praise your spouse for working out or just looking good. Acknowledge the progress they've made—even if it's small. Everyone wants to feel good, and offering a compliment here and there acts as a much better motivator than any kind of criticism or judgment.

➤ Do offer forbidden foods from time to time, like a slice of cake or a homemade oatmeal cookie. Not allowing these things often has the opposite effect than you've intended. When they know you're not judging them for eating something sweet, it can lead to less sneaking around or making the better decision on their own.

➤ When it comes to your kids, moms are the CEOs of the family and must try to keep everyone in shape, healthy and doing well. But do your best to let your kids make their own decisions without coming down too hard on them. Your children have learned their habits from watching you, so the best defense is a good offense—be a great role model with your food choices and exercise routines.

➤ Do not let your daughters hear you complaining about your weight—ever. What they see, they do, and you don't want them developing poor body image or eating issues.

➤ If you aren't feeling good about yourself, don't play it out in front of the kids because they will begin their own pattern of self-deprecation.

➤ Don't come down on your kids for eating because you want to be helpful. Your criticism is not what they need to hear.

➤ Do encourage your kids to find activities that get them outside and away from the TV or video games. Try doing something active together as a family, such as a hike, a bike ride or a run.

CHAPTER THIRTEEN

The Kids Are Not All Right

Recent studies have shown that 47 percent of girls in the fifth through twelfth grades want to lose weight because of pictures they see in magazines.

Sixty-nine percent of girls in the fifth through twelfth grade admit that pictures in magazines influenced their idea of a perfect body shape.

Forty-two percent of first through third grade girls want to be thinner.

Eighty-one percent of ten year olds are afraid of being fat.

Ninety-five percent of those who have eating disorders are between the ages of twelve and twenty-five.

The number of obese children and teens in the United States continues to grow at alarming rates. An incredible 30 percent of American children are either overweight or obese and have an 80 percent chance of becoming overweight adults. Obesity in children can lead to chronic problems later in life including heart disease, hypertension, high cholesterol, high blood pressure, Type 2 diabetes, asthma, knee and joint problems, sleep apnea and a life span that can be shortened by up to fourteen years, just to name a few. And, scariest of all, overweight children are more likely to grow up to become overweight weathermen.

Of course, the worst part of being a heavy kid isn't the possibility of bad health; it's the ridicule and social discrimination that takes place. The psychological stress of teasing and ostracizing usually leads to low self-esteem, which can have long-term damaging effects on everything from their schoolwork to their social lives. Being a teenager is hard enough without being a teenager who feels bad about the way he or she looks. It's tough enough to be a grown woman trying to navigate the treacherous world of women's magazines, size zero clothing and the endless weight loss ads, let alone a prepubescent or teenage girl!

Girls as young as seven years old are now being treated for anorexia and girls as young as three and four years old wish they were thinner. Girls, especially overweight girls, get so many negative messages about their bodies in our culture, and that makes it even harder for them to live up to the media's expectations. When it comes to weight, a lot of parents, especially dads, aren't sure how to talk to their kids about weight because it can be a highly sensitive subject.

My dad was the consummate father. He was a teacher, a friend, a buddy and, yes, a disciplinarian. After I became a father, I came to really appreciate what he did for all of his kids along the way. I could understand why he worked back-to-back shifts as a bus driver and why he worked all of those odd jobs on the side. Some people might say being out of the house was the only way he could get any peace and quiet. But I know better. It was because he wanted the best for his children. And that is what any dad wants for his kids—including me, especially when it comes to their health and well-being.

Genetically speaking, my daughter Leila takes after me while our son, Nicky, tends to be more like his mother. What this means is that Leila is going to have to work a little harder on keeping her weight in a healthy place than her brother will have to, even more so because Nicky has always been more into physical activities such as tae kwon do, running and biking.

Kids develop their eating habits and attitude toward food from their parents. If parents go to fast food restaurants and expose their kids to lots of junk food, children will develop those same habits, which are extremely hard to break. To be the best example for your kids you have to do more than what you say. You have to lead by example. Even if you haven't always made the healthiest choices in the past, it's never too late to develop new healthy habits. To do this, slowly remove the less healthy foods from your house and start replacing them with healthy alternatives such as low-fat yogurt, fresh fruit, raw veggies, hummus, whole grain cereals, pasta and breads, and lean meat and poultry. Make it easy for yourself to make healthy meals anytime.

While it's important to establish healthy eating habits, I believe it's equally important not to deprive your children of special treats from time to time. The key to their success is allowing them choices while teaching moderation. Your children will encounter temptation in the real world, so you have to give them the ability to make good decisions. Depriving them of the things they see their friends eating will only encourage them to overindulge in your absence, setting them up to become binge eaters. (Remember my cereal story from college?)

· ·

Improving your lifestyle can inspire your overweight child to do the same. It's great for kids to see their parents changing their eating habits and getting more exercise. I had my gastric bypass surgery when Leila was just three years old, so she doesn't really remember me as "fat dad." She will look at pictures from before my weight loss and simply say, "You look so different." Nicky was born shortly after I'd lost one hundred pounds, so he has never known me any other way. He looks at old pictures of me and thinks it's someone else.

I had always sworn that when I became a father, I would be a cool dad. I wouldn't use those tired old sayings that have been passed on from generation to generation in my family. You know the ones. "When I was your age, I knew the value of a dollar," and "Sorry won't do your homework, walk the dog or put the garbage out, will it!" So far, I've done pretty well at avoiding those statements! But there have been a few times I said things I wish I hadn't—especially when it comes to food.

At least I made it a point never to use food as a reward or a source of comfort for my children, because I am well aware of what that path leads to. But I know how hard it is to talk to your kids honestly about their weight, even if they ask you about it! The best course is to be available to help and support them on their own journey, without being their conscience.

Because I worry about my children, I sometimes have to catch myself when I see Leila heading to the dessert table for a second time or when she orders pasta for dinner for the third time that week. Saying something or judging your kid is a slippery slope for any parent. No teenager on the planet wants their parents to ask, "Are you sure you want to eat that?" or "Haven't you had enough?" I know this because I am a grown man and I still can't tolerate someone saying those things to me. Anytime I'm tempted to react, I remind myself how that made me feel. I don't want to make Leila feel guilty or uptight about food any more than I want her to go to the places I've been in my personal struggle. It's something I need to guard myself against or risk hurting her in ways that I never meant.

I grew up the target of chubby jokes so I know the pain and the shame that comes with that. As a parent, I want to protect my children from anything that could bring them harm, yet I have to remind myself not to go overboard trying to protect my kids from the same trap I fell into because it's their journey—not mine.

Surprisingly, it is my teenage daughter who taught me one of the most valuable lessons I've ever learned about women. She doesn't want me to solve her problems. She just wants to know she can come and talk to me and make sure I hear her.

"Hello. I am Dr. Frasier Crane and I am listening . . ."

She's not looking for me to comment (unless she asks for my take, and even then, I need to be cautious; she might not want to hear what I really think). She just wants to talk, be heard and feel acknowledged without me being logical or judgmental or giving her advice. Thank you, Leila, for teaching your old man such an important life lesson.

One of the ways I connect with my kids to positively reinforce their health and fitness is by participating in projects and sports together. My older daughter, Courtney, just graduated from culinary school, so she and I have a great time experimenting in the kitchen together, trying new foods, adjusting favorite family recipes to make them healthier and making up our own creations. Leila has recently taken an interest in going to the gym. I am really proud of her for coming to this decision on her own. I support her by doing whatever I can to make it easy for her to go, and I praise her and tell her how focused she is on her health. She's not only running and doing weights, she's taking Pilates and yoga. You go, girl.

Nicky loves to ride his bike and go for runs, so this is always a great way for us to spend some quality father-son time together. When the four of us are all together, Debra and I will make it a point to plan some kind of activity we can do as a family such as a hike or a bike ride, especially when we're on vacation.

Your long-term goal as a parent is to raise children who know they're loved and who are comfortable with who they are regardless of their size. Helping them build a better body image is just as critical as building strong self-esteem. Kids need to know that what you feel about them has nothing to do with their weight, that your love is not based on what they eat or don't eat. If your children know they are loved and can learn to love themselves no matter what, they are likely to make healthy choices along the way. That's one of the greatest gifts you could ever pass on to your children.

CHAPTER FOURTEEN

Stop the Insanity

Albert Einstein once said that the definition of insanity is "doing the same thing over and over again and expecting different results." Boy, if this is true, I went nuts a long time ago! But somewhere along the way I came to my senses and realized I had to make a choice: keep living the same way I'd been living and spend the rest of my life on a roller-coaster ride I'd never get off, or get real and make some drastic changes in lifestyle that would likely prolong if not save my life altogether.

What's holding you back?

What excuses are you making up that are stopping you from living your best life?

By now you know I used them all, and look where that circle jerk got me!

Chasing my tail like a puppy that ran around and around and never got what he was looking for!

Are you ready to stop the craziness and get real with yourself?

••

If so, it's time to take a look at what your life really looks like. Hey, I'm just the guy who is willing to hold up the mirror for you. If you don't like what you see, don't break the mirror—*make a change.*

Take a serious look at your eating habits. Are you really aware of what you're putting in your mouth every day? You would probably be shocked at what you found if you kept track. Start writing down everything you eat for the next couple of weeks and see if that meshes with what you thought you were eating. So many of us eat without being conscious of what we are doing, eating more out of *habit* than *hunger.*

Guess what.

That's why you're fat!

It took me years to understand that *hunger fades.* You don't need to eat the second you feel that rumble in your stomach. Wait it out. See what happens in twenty minutes or so. Chances are, you aren't hungry so much as you are bored. Look, I was that guy who grabbed for something to eat the second my stomach grumbled or I had a couple of spare minutes with nothing to do, or I was going through something traumatic and food made me feel better or, or, or . . . I didn't really need a reason. The bottom line was that it was easy to mindlessly eat, but it never made me feel good. When you change your awareness of food and become a conscious eater, you will see that eating healthy is a *choice.* You have the option to choose an apple or a chocolate chip muffin. It's not that hard, but it does take putting yourself in the right mind-set to get there. If you're not ready or you're doing it for someone else, you will fail.

Rule #1: You must do this for you.
Rule #2: See Rule #1.

●●

The next thing you need to do is take an inventory of your level of activity. How much are you really moving every day? And no, getting up from your favorite chair or cozy sofa to grab a bite to eat from the kitchen does not count as exercise!

Get up and move!

Take a walk around your neighborhood, start biking in the park, join a gym, start swimming laps at the local community pool or find a sport that you've been "meaning" to get back to or take up and just do it. You don't have to train for a marathon to get into the mind-set of an athlete. You just need the *desire* to be active, the *discipline* to follow through and the *motivation* to stick with it. You don't even have to enjoy it, but it helps. And besides, what's the alternative?

To stay a couch potato for the rest of your life?

I don't think so!

As we age, our metabolism slows down and therefore we have to do more to keep it revved. Eating a healthy, clean diet and participating in a mild exercise program are the keys to your success. The pounds will not only come off, they will stay off. When you change your lifestyle, you change your life. It's really that simple.

I've thought a lot about my dad since his passing many years ago and have asked myself if he would have approved of my decision to have the gastric bypass surgery to finally lose the weight I'd been carrying around for so many years. In the end, I think he would have been pleased with my decision and very proud of the work I've put into keeping it off for more than a decade now. I can sometimes hear him say, "You did good, Albert, but don't get cocky!"

I occasionally fear slipping back. I think everyone who has ever been where I've been and who is constantly struggling with their weight feels the same way. I still think about food about as often as the average male thinks about sex—which is about every ten seconds or so. But sex can be a great motivator, because if I had to choose between that Krispy Kreme donut or sex with my wife, I'm going with the sex!

Actually, sex with Deborah *while eating a Krispy Kreme donut* would be amazing!

Still, ever since I was a kid I've thought about what my next meal would be, and when I got older, what I would make for dinner—even if I was still eating breakfast! I don't think this will ever change, but my approach to food and eating definitely has. I know I won't get paralyzed by fear, change or the unknown—in fact, I use all of it as my motivation to keep making the right choices that are good for my health. I now understand firsthand what it is like to live as a fit and trim man, and I appreciate the happiness and freedom my newfound health has brought to my life. I now have the ability to see a pint of ice cream, have a single spoonful and walk away. With some foods, not having any is easier than having only one bite. The point is to have control over food instead of food controlling you.

My weight will continue to be a lifelong battle, but at least I'm prepared to face it head-on and slay the dragon. I know it'll take hard work, discipline, perseverance and persistence. If I had a choice between going on a twelve-mile run or sitting at home in front of the fire and reading a book, in my heart, I would prefer the book, but I am aware that isn't going to keep me in shape. So when I look at the alternatives and weigh the options, there's one thing I know for sure—I no longer identify myself as the fat, jolly, rotund weatherman. That guy is gone. It doesn't mean he won't try to stage a comeback. But if he does, I'm ready for him, because I love where I am, and I'm never goin' back!

Recipes

The following recipes are excellent examples of how well you can eat while eating clean. Developed by Melissa Bowman Li for her clients, these recipes are simple to make, delicious and will keep you looking great. Once you start eating this way, you will find it's not hard to follow and, best of all, you will look and feel great.

BREAKFAST

Egg Scramble (Vegetarian)

(1 serving)

INGREDIENTS:

- 1 whole egg
- 3 egg whites
- sea salt and pepper, to taste
- 1 tbsp extra-virgin olive oil
- 2 tbsp scallions, sliced
- ¼ cup tomatoes, diced
- ¼ avocado, diced

INSTRUCTIONS:

1. Whisk egg and egg whites together in a medium bowl until well combined.

2. Season with some sea salt and pepper and add a splash of water.

3. Bring a medium sauté pan to medium heat with olive oil.

4. Add eggs to the pan and allow them to set a bit before stirring.

5. Once your eggs are beginning to cook, sprinkle in the scallions and tomatoes and gently fold all the ingredients into your eggs. Cook through.

6. Top the egg scramble with diced avocado.

Breakfast Burrito (Vegetarian)

(1 serving)

INGREDIENTS:

1 tsp grape seed oil	3 egg whites
¼ cup onion, diced	1 whole egg
½ red pepper, diced	1 tbsp cilantro, chopped
sea salt and pepper, to taste	1 rice tortilla
¼ tsp cumin	¼ avocado, diced

INSTRUCTIONS:

1. Heat grape seed oil in a skillet and add onion and pepper. Sauté for 5 minutes, until your vegetables are tender.

2. Season with sea salt, pepper and cumin.

3. Stir in your egg and scramble everything together.

4. Cook for 3–4 minutes. Right before your eggs are set, stir in the cilantro.

5. Shut off the heat and allow the eggs to finish cooking from the heat of the pan.

6. In the meantime, heat your tortilla up by placing it right over a burner with a low heat. Give it about 20 seconds or so on each side until it is warmed through and slightly charred (you can also heat the tortilla up in the oven on low heat).

7. Fill tortilla with the scramble and top with freshly diced avocado.

8. Cut in half and serve.

Plain Quinoa (Vegetarian)

(4 servings)

INGREDIENTS:

1 cup raw quinoa, rinsed well
2 cups purified water, vegetable broth or chicken broth
pinch of sea salt

INSTRUCTIONS:

1. Place quinoa, water or broth and sea salt in a medium saucepan. Bring to a boil.

2. Turn the heat to low, cover and allow it to simmer for about 15 minutes.

3. When the quinoa is done, it will be translucent and have a little white circle around it (that's the germ).

4. If you want your quinoa to take on a nuttier flavor, dry roast it in a skillet for a few minutes before cooking.

Quinoa Breakfast (Vegetarian)

(1 serving)

INGREDIENTS:

- ¼ cup raw quinoa, rinsed well
- ½ cup unsweetened rice, coconut or almond milk
- 2 tsp raw walnuts
- ½ cup blueberries or raspberries
- sprinkle of cinnamon and/or nutmeg

INSTRUCTIONS:

1. Combine quinoa and milk in a small saucepan and place over medium to low heat.

2. Once the mixture comes to a boil, turn it down to a simmer.

3. Allow it to cook for about 5 minutes, until the porridge has thickened and is heated through.

4. Stir in walnuts and fruit. Top with cinnamon and nutmeg.

Egg Sauté (Vegetarian)

(1 serving)

INGREDIENTS:

1 tbsp extra-virgin olive oil
¼ cup red onion, minced
1 handful kale, chopped
⅓ cup canned black beans
2–3 egg whites
1 whole egg
1 roma tomato, diced
sea salt and pepper, to taste

INSTRUCTIONS:

1. In a sauté pan with the olive oil, cook the onions until they begin to become transparent.

2. Add the kale and beans, cooking until the kale leaves darken, soften and are shiny.

3. Add eggs and cook thoroughly while stirring mixture.

4. Top with diced tomato.

5. Season with sea salt and pepper.

*Wrap in a rice tortilla for breakfast on the go.

Fresh Vegetable Omelet Muffins
(Vegetarian)

(6 servings)

INGREDIENTS:

6 whole eggs, beaten
sea salt and pepper, to taste
coconut oil
1–2 cups of desired vegetables, diced. (You can use any vegetables. My favorite combo is red bell peppers, jalapeño peppers and cilantro!)
¼ cup sugar-free salsa (optional)

INSTRUCTIONS:

1. Preheat oven to 350°F.

2. Season beaten eggs with sea salt and pepper.

3. Lightly coat a 6-cup muffin pan with coconut oil (use a paper towel to spread evenly).

4. Divide vegetables evenly into each of the 6 muffin pan slots.

5. Fill each muffin slot with the egg batter.

6. Bake for 20–25 minutes until set.

Rice and Eggs (Vegetarian)

(1 serving)

INGREDIENTS:

> 2 eggs
> ½ cup cooked brown or wild rice
> 1 tsp extra-virgin olive oil
> sea salt and pepper, to taste

INSTRUCTIONS:

1. Sauté eggs in olive oil, sunny side up.

2. Top cooked rice with eggs.

3. Season with sea salt and pepper.

LUNCH/DINNER

Turkey and Avocado Sandwich

(1 serving)

INGREDIENTS:

> ½ cup lettuce
> 3–4 oz cooked turkey breast
> ¼ avocado
> sea salt
> 1 slice of gluten-free bread

INSTRUCTIONS:

1. Layer ingredients on bread and serve.

••

Tuna Salad

(1 serving)

INGREDIENTS:

6 oz can wild caught tuna, drained and flaked
¼ cup red pepper, chopped
1 celery stalk, chopped
1 tsp lemon juice
sea salt and pepper, to taste
rice crackers (optional)

INSTRUCTIONS:

1. Mix together tuna, pepper, celery and lemon juice.

2. Season with sea salt and pepper.

3. Serve with rice crackers.

*If you want to omit the rice crackers, this tuna salad can also be served over a green salad.

Cucumber Tuna Boats

(3 servings)

INGREDIENTS:

3 medium cucumbers
6 oz can wild caught tuna, drained and flaked
2 hard-boiled eggs, chopped
½ cup celery, diced
1 tbsp onion, finely chopped
1 tsp lemon juice
sea salt and pepper, to taste

INSTRUCTIONS:

1. Peel the cucumbers and cut in half lengthwise. Remove and discard the seeds.

2. In a bowl, combine the remaining ingredients. Spoon into the cucumber boats. Serve immediately.

Quinoa with Poached Egg, Spinach and Cucumber (Vegetarian)

(2 servings)

INGREDIENTS:

3 tbsp extra-virgin olive oil
1 garlic clove, sliced
5 oz spinach, rinsed
sea salt, to taste
1 carrot, julienned
2 eggs

1 cup cooked quinoa
  (see page 189)
¼ cucumber, thinly sliced
1 tsp rice vinegar
red chili flakes, to taste
1 tsp chives, minced

INSTRUCTIONS:

1. Heat 1 tbsp olive oil in a skillet over medium heat.

2. Add sliced garlic clove and cook for 1 minute.

3. Add the spinach and steam, covered, until wilted (about 1 minute).

4. Season with sea salt and transfer to a plate.

5. Rinse the pan and fill with 2 inches water; bring to a boil.

6. Add the carrot and cook until tender (about 1 minute); transfer to a plate.

7. Reduce heat to a simmer and poach the eggs for 3–4 minutes.

8. Divide the quinoa between each bowl, top with egg, spinach, carrot and cucumber.

9. Whisk the rice vinegar, remaining olive oil and sea salt together, drizzling over the bowls.

10. Sprinkle with red chili flakes and minced chives.

Bean and Vegetable Pasta (Vegetarian)

(2 servings)

INGREDIENTS:

8 oz canned white beans (pea, navy, great northern)
1 onion, chopped
1 carrot, chopped
½ tsp dried oregano
1 tbsp dried basil
1 tbsp extra-virgin olive oil
8 oz canned tomatoes
¼ cup bean liquid
1 tsp sea salt
pepper, to taste
¼ lb rice elbow macaroni

INSTRUCTIONS:

1. Drain beans, reserving liquid.

2. Sauté the onions, carrots, oregano and basil in olive oil.

3. Add tomatoes, bean liquid, sea salt and pepper.

4. Cover and simmer for about 10 minutes, until the vegetables are tender.

5. Add the drained beans and simmer for another 10 minutes.

6. Meanwhile, cook and drain the macaroni.

7. Toss cooked pasta with more olive oil and then mix with the bean sauce.

Veggie "Mac & Cheese" (Vegetarian)

(4 servings)

INGREDIENTS:

1 small butternut squash, peeled, seeded and diced
1 carrot, chopped
½ lb brown rice macaroni
½ cup unsweetened almond milk
sea salt and pepper, to taste

INSTRUCTIONS:

1. Steam squash and carrot until soft.

2. Meanwhile, cook and drain rice macaroni.

3. Puree squash and carrot with the almond milk.

4. Add sea salt and pepper, to taste.

5. Add sauce to noodles and serve.

Chicken Bean Quesadilla

(4 servings)

INGREDIENTS:

2 tbsp extra-virgin olive oil
2 rice tortillas
2 chicken breasts, grilled and
    diced into chunks
16 oz canned black beans

Additional filling ideas:
red onion
bell peppers
jalapeño peppers
tomatoes
chillies

Topping ideas:
salsa
guacamole
pico de gallo (tomato, red
    onion, jalapeño, lime
    juice, cilantro, sea
    salt and pepper)
lettuce

INSTRUCTIONS:

1. Preheat oven to 350°F.

2. Line a baking sheet with tinfoil and mist with olive oil.

3. Place one tortilla on prepared baking sheet.

4. Top with chicken, black beans and desired fillings.

5. Place second tortilla on top.

6. Mist top tortilla with olive oil. Bake for 18 minutes.

7. Turn on broiler and broil for 2–3 minutes or until tortilla is browned.

8. Cut in quarters, add toppings if desired and serve.

Chicken Margarita Pizza

(2–3 servings)

INGREDIENTS:

- 1 gluten- and sugar-free pizza crust (Namaste Foods pizza crust mix)
- 1 garlic clove
- 2 tbsp extra-virgin olive oil
- 2 tomatoes, sliced
- basil leaves
- 1 chicken breast, cooked and shredded
- sea salt and pepper, to taste
- *Other toppings to try out include bell peppers, jalapeño peppers, onion and fresh herbs!

INSTRUCTIONS:

1. Preheat oven to 400°F.
2. Rub crust with garlic clove and olive oil.
3. Layer with tomato, basil and chicken (or other desired "clean" toppings).
4. Season with sea salt and pepper.
5. Bake till heated (7–10 minutes).

Crunchy Chicken Wraps

(1 serving)

INGREDIENTS:

1 chicken breast
4 romaine lettuce leaves
¼ cup cucumber, sliced
¼ cup radishes, sliced
¼ cup sprouts
1 tbsp lemon juice

INSTRUCTIONS:

1. Grill chicken breast and cut into slices.

2. Layer romaine lettuce leaves with sliced cucumber and sliced radish.

3. Layer on chicken.

4. Top with sprouts and a bit of lemon juice.

5. Fold up lettuce over ingredients and enjoy!

Grilled Chicken and Vegetable Kebabs

(1 serving)

INGREDIENTS:

1 chicken breast, cut into chunks
½ cup cherry tomatoes
½ cup bell peppers, cut into cubes
½ cup white or red onion, cut into cubes
1 tbsp extra-virgin olive oil
1 tbsp balsamic vinegar
sea salt and pepper, to taste

INSTRUCTIONS:

1. Skewer ingredients, alternating the chicken, tomatoes, peppers and onion.

2. Rub with olive oil and vinegar, and season with sea salt and pepper.

3. Grill until chicken is fully cooked.

*These can also be cooked in the oven.

Garlic and Basil Chicken with Tomato Salsa

(4 servings)

INGREDIENTS:

For the chicken:

½ cup fresh basil leaves
3 garlic cloves
¼ cup extra-virgin olive oil
sea salt and pepper, to taste
4 chicken breasts

For the salsa:

2 cups rainbow cherry/grape tomatoes, halved
½ cup fresh basil leaves, chopped
¼ cup extra-virgin olive oil
¼ cup balsamic vinegar
1 garlic clove, minced
sea salt and pepper, to taste

INSTRUCTIONS:

1. Make the chicken rub: Blend basil, garlic, olive oil, sea salt and pepper in food processor until roughly chopped.

2. Rub over chicken.

3. Make the salsa: Mix together the above salsa ingredients and leave to stand for 30 minutes.

4. Grill the chicken until thoroughly cooked; allow to rest for 5 minutes.

5. Spoon salsa over chicken to serve.

• •

Sage, Chicken and Apples

(4 servings)

INGREDIENTS:

- 4 chicken breasts
- extra-virgin olive oil
- sea salt and pepper, to taste
- 1 tbsp sage, chopped
- 3 apples, cored and quartered
- 1 onion, cut into large chunks
- ⅔ cup unsweetened apple juice

INSTRUCTIONS:

1. Preheat oven to 425°F.

2. Season chicken with olive oil, sea salt, pepper and sage. Lightly brown all sides in a sauté pan.

3. Transfer chicken and juices to a small roasting pan and add the rest of the ingredients.

4. Bake for 15–20 minutes or until internal temperature is 155°F.

5. Rest for 10 minutes.

Coconut Lime Chicken

(4 servings)

INGREDIENTS:

4 chicken breasts
3 tbsp lime juice (or more as needed)
½ cup unsweetened coconut milk
sea salt, to taste
2 tbsp lime zest
1 pinch cayenne pepper
¼ cup green onions, chopped
1 handful cilantro, chopped

INSTRUCTIONS:

1. Marinate chicken in 1½ tbsp lime juice.

2. Grill chicken.

3. Warm coconut milk over low heat.

4. Season the coconut milk with sea salt, lime zest and cayenne pepper.

5. Add the remaining lime juice to coconut mixture.

6. Pour sauce over chicken and garnish with green onions and cilantro.

7. Squeeze remaining lime juice over finished dish, if desired.

Chicken and Balsamic Peppers

(4 servings)

INGREDIENTS:

4 large bell peppers (red, green, orange, yellow); cored and sliced thin

1 large sweet onion, sliced

⅓ cup balsamic vinegar

¼ cup extra-virgin olive oil

¼ cup chicken broth

6 garlic cloves, chopped

1 tbsp dried basil

½ tsp dried thyme

½ tsp dried rosemary

4 chicken breasts, split

sea salt and pepper, to taste

INSTRUCTIONS:

1. Preheat oven to 375°F.

2. Toss the pepper and onion slices in a large bowl.

3. In a large measuring cup, whisk your dressing of balsamic vinegar, olive oil, broth, chopped garlic and herbs.

4. Pour the sauce over the sliced peppers, onions and toss well to coat.

5. Place the split chicken breasts in the bottom of a baking pan sprayed with olive oil.

6. Season with sea salt and pepper, to taste.

7. Pour the balsamic pepper dressing over the chicken and arrange them evenly.

8. Loosely cover the pan with a piece of foil and place in the center of a preheated oven.

9. Bake for 45–60 minutes until chicken is cooked through and peppers are soft.

Chicken Tacos with Guacamole

(2 servings)

INGREDIENTS:

8 oz ground chicken
2 tsp extra-virgin olive oil
½ onion, chopped
¼ cup purified water
½ tomato, chopped
1 radicchio lettuce head

For the taco seasoning:

1 tbsp chili powder
2 tbsp garlic powder
¼ tsp dried oregano
½ tsp paprika
2 tsp ground cumin
1 tsp sea salt

For the guacamole:

1 avocado
½ onion, chopped
¼ cup cilantro (plus 1 tbsp
    for garnish), chopped
½ tomato, chopped
juice of 1 lime
¼ tsp cumin
¼ tsp white pepper
1 garlic clove
1 tsp sea salt

INSTRUCTIONS:

1. Sauté chicken in olive oil until white. Add onion.

2. Combine ingredients for taco seasoning and stir in.

3. Stir in water and bring to boil, simmer for 10 minutes. Add chopped tomato.

4. Prepare guacamole by adding all ingredients together and blending until combined. Chill in fridge.

5. Prepare radicchio leaves by cutting off the bottom and separating the leaves to make the "taco shells."

6. Top the shells with taco meat, guacamole and additional cilantro.

••

Chicken Ragout

(4 servings)

INGREDIENTS:

    4 chicken breasts, cut into chunks
    2 tbsp extra-virgin olive oil
    2 garlic cloves, minced
    1 small zucchini, halved and cut into thick slices
    2 tomatoes, chopped
    ½ tsp thyme
    ½ tsp oregano
    sea salt and pepper, to taste

INSTRUCTIONS:

1. In a large skillet over medium heat, sauté chicken in olive oil for 2–3 minutes.

2. Add remaining ingredients and sauté for 5 minutes, stirring once or twice.

3. Cover with a lid, turn heat down to low and simmer for 10–12 minutes.

Ratatouille with Brown Rice (Vegetarian)

(6 servings)

INGREDIENTS:

2 large onions, sliced

3 garlic cloves, minced

½ cup extra-virgin olive oil

1 medium eggplant, cut into chunks

2 green peppers, chopped

3 zucchini, cut into slices

1 tsp oregano

½ tsp thyme

¼ tsp pepper

sea salt, to taste

28 oz canned tomatoes, drained, or 4 cups fresh tomatoes, chopped

6 servings of brown rice, cooked

INSTRUCTIONS:

1. In a large pot, sauté onion and garlic in olive oil for 2 minutes.

2. Add eggplant and sauté for 5 minutes.

3. Add peppers and cook for 5 minutes.

4. Add zucchini and cook for 5 minutes; then add seasonings and tomatoes.

5. Cover and simmer for 30 minutes.

6. Serve ratatouille with brown rice.

Chili (Vegetarian)

(4–6 servings)

INGREDIENTS:

2 medium onions, diced
4 garlic cloves, minced
2 medium peppers, diced
1 tbsp extra-virgin olive oil
28 oz canned Italian tomatoes (reserve juice)
2 cups purified water
15 oz canned pinto or kidney beans, drained
1–2 tbsp chili powder
1 jalapeño pepper, finely chopped (optional for extra spice)
½ tsp cumin
¼ tsp pepper
sea salt, to taste
¼ cup buckwheat groats

INSTRUCTIONS:

1. In a large skillet, sauté onions, garlic and peppers in olive oil. Add tomatoes (and tomato juice).

2. Add water, beans and spices.

3. Bring to a boil, stir and cover.

4. Reduce heat and simmer for 10–15 minutes.

5. Add buckwheat groats and cook covered for 10–15 minutes more or until the groats are tender.

6. Taste and adjust seasoning if desired.

7. Serve hot.

••

Chicken Chili

(2 servings)

INGREDIENTS:

1 onion, diced
2 tbsp extra-virgin olive oil
1 red bell pepper, cut into chunks
1 cup canned Italian tomatoes
1 cup chicken broth
1 tsp dried chili flakes
1 tsp dried oregano
2 chicken breasts, diced
1 cup canned red kidney beans
fresh coriander
1 tbsp lime juice
½ avocado, sliced

INSTRUCTIONS:

1. Heat oven to 350°F.
2. Sauté the onions in olive oil until soft; add in the peppers, canned tomatoes, chicken broth, chili and oregano. Stir.
3. Add the diced chicken breast, making sure it is covered in the sauce.
4. Bring to a simmer and then cook in the oven for 40 minutes.
5. Add the red kidney beans and bake for another 20 minutes.
6. Serve piping hot and season with coriander and lime juice. Top with sliced avocado.

••

Turkey Chili

(10 servings)

INGREDIENTS:

1 large red onion, chopped

1 large green bell pepper, chopped

6 garlic cloves, diced

1 tbsp extra-virgin olive oil

1½ lbs lean ground turkey meat

4 tbsp ground cumin

1 tsp ground coriander

1 tbsp chili powder

1 vegetable bouillon cube (gluten-free), dissolved in 1 cup purified water

3 cups fresh tomatoes, diced

6 oz canned tomato paste (no sugar added)

15 oz canned kidney beans

15 oz canned tomato sauce (no sugar added) (optional)

2–3 scallions, chopped (for garnish)

INSTRUCTIONS:

1. In a large soup pot, sauté the red onion, bell pepper and garlic cloves in olive oil until the onions become translucent.

2. Add the turkey meat and continue to stir until the meat is cooked.

3. Stir in cumin, coriander and chili powder.

4. Pour in the water with the dissolved bouillon cube.

5. Add the tomatoes, tomato paste and beans.

6. Keep at a low and steady boil for about 5–10 minutes to allow the spices to really absorb.

7. If you find the chili is too thick or dry, add the can of tomato sauce.

8. Cool and serve. Garnish with chopped scallions.

• •

Veggie Burgers (Vegetarian)

(8 servings)

INGREDIENTS:

2 tsp extra-virgin olive oil
1 small bell pepper, diced
¼ cup celery, diced
1 tbsp parsley
1 tsp thyme
½ tsp pepper
pinch of cayenne pepper
½ tsp sea salt
1½ cups cooked lentils
4 egg whites
¼ cup sunflower seeds

INSTRUCTIONS:

1. In a sauté pan, combine olive oil, bell pepper, celery and spices for 5 minutes.

2. Combine this mixture with the rest of the ingredients in a food processor.

3. Pulse until ingredients begin to clump.

4. Form mixture into 8 patties.

5. Sauté veggie burger patties in olive oil until egg whites are cooked through. Serve warm.

Turkey and Guacamole Burgers

(6 servings)

INGREDIENTS:

For the guacamole:

2 avocados
1 tsp garlic powder
½ tsp black pepper
2 jalapeños, finely chopped
½ white onion, finely chopped
1 cup cilantro, finely chopped
juice of 1 lime

For the burgers:

2 lbs lean ground turkey
4 tsp ground cinnamon
1 tsp garlic powder
1 tsp black pepper
extra-virgin olive oil
iceberg lettuce, 1 whole leaf per
    burger, washed and dried

INSTRUCTIONS:

For the guacamole:

1. Cut avocados in half. Remove the pits and scoop flesh into a medium-size bowl.

2. Add garlic powder, black pepper, jalapeños, white onions, cilantro and lime juice.

3. Mix all ingredients together (do not overmix). Chill before serving.

For the burgers:

1. Preheat your grill or grill pan to medium-high heat.

2. Add turkey, cinnamon, garlic powder and black pepper to a large bowl. Mix together with clean bare hands.

3. Divide the mixture into 6 parts and mold into flat patties.

4. Lightly coat the hot grill with olive oil and add the patties.

5. Grill patties for 7–9 minutes on each side, until cooked through.

6. Top each burger with guacamole and wrap in iceberg lettuce leaves.

••

Halibut in Parchment

(1 serving)

INGREDIENTS:

1 small fennel bulb, sliced
sea salt and pepper, to taste
1 halibut fillet
herbes de Provence (lavender, fennel, basil, thyme)
2 tbsp extra-virgin olive oil
1 lemon slice

INSTRUCTIONS:

1. Preheat oven to 400°F.

2. Cut one 8" x 12" piece each of parchment and foil.

3. Place parchment on foil and center fennel slices on the paper.

4. Season with sea salt and pepper.

5. Place the halibut fillet on top; season with sea salt and pepper.

6. Sprinkle with herbes de Provence.

7. Drizzle with olive oil.

8. Pull the long side of the parchment up to the center, overlapping to a close and fold back the ends under the packet.

9. Bake on a cookie sheet at 400°F for 6–8 minutes until the packet puffs up with steam.

10. Serve with a lemon wheel.

Chili Lime Tilapia Pouches

(4 servings)

INGREDIENTS:

- juice of 1 lime
- 1 tbsp chili powder
- 1 tsp cayenne pepper
- 2 shallots, thinly sliced
- 1 package fresh spinach
- 4 tilapia fillets

INSTRUCTIONS:

1. Preheat the oven to 375°F.

2. In a small bowl, mix lime juice, chili powder, cayenne pepper and shallots.

3. Place spinach leaves on a large rectangle of foil, then add tilapia fillets. Spoon the lime juice mixture over the fish. Fold the foil up and roll edges to create an airtight pouch.

4. Cook in preheated 375°F oven for about 15 minutes (cooking time will vary depending on oven temperature and how many pieces of fish you are cooking).

Almond-Crusted Salmon

(2 servings)

INGREDIENTS:

½ cup raw almonds
sea salt and pepper, to taste
2 salmon fillets
2 tsp extra-virgin olive oil
1 lemon

INSTRUCTIONS:

1. Preheat oven to 350°F.

2. Crush almonds to small pieces in a sandwich bag with sea salt and pepper.

3. Pat salmon dry with a paper towel, cover with a light coating of olive oil and the almond topping.

4. Bake skin side down, uncovered for 10–15 minutes.

5. Squeeze lemon juice over fish and season with sea salt and pepper.

Steamed Salmon with Herbs and Lemon

(1 serving)

INGREDIENTS:

1 salmon fillet
sea salt and pepper,
to taste

fresh herbs (dill, parsley,
chives), chopped
zest of 1 lemon

INSTRUCTIONS:

1. Season salmon with sea salt and pepper.

2. Steam until just cooked through (7–8 minutes).

3. Sprinkle with fresh chopped herbs and lemon zest.

SALAD RECIPES

Green Salad (Vegetarian)

(2–3 servings)

INGREDIENTS:

3 cups mixed greens
1 cup cucumber, chopped
1 cup radishes, chopped

½ cup red onion, finely
chopped

INSTRUCTIONS:

1. Combine mixed greens with chopped cucumber, radishes and red onion.

2. Drizzle with basic salad dressing.

• •

Clean Salad Dressing

INGREDIENTS:

¼ cup flaxseed oil or 2 tbsp each flaxseed and olive oil
1–2 tbsp balsamic vinegar
1 tbsp purified water
whole or minced garlic, herbs (e.g., oregano, basil)

INSTRUCTIONS:

1. Mix basic salad dressing ingredients in shaker jar and store any leftovers in your refrigerator.

2. Increase recipe for multiple servings.

Raw Kale Salad with Pomegranate and Toasted Walnuts (Vegetarian)

(4 servings)

INGREDIENTS:

1 bunch kale, torn
2 tbsp extra-virgin olive oil
1 tbsp fresh lime juice
½ tsp ginger, peeled and grated

½ cup pomegranate seeds
2 tbsp red onion, chopped
¼ cup toasted walnuts, chopped
sea salt and pepper, to taste

INSTRUCTIONS:

1. Rub torn kale with olive oil, lime juice and grated ginger until well coated.

2. Add the pomegranate seeds, red onion and walnuts. Toss together.

3. Season with sea salt and pepper.

••

Roasted Vegetable Quinoa Salad (Vegetarian)

(4–5 servings)

INGREDIENTS:

- 1 medium zucchini, chopped
- 1 medium carrot, chopped
- 1 small red onion, chopped
- 2 cups cooked quinoa
- 2 cups purified water
- juice of 1 lemon
- sea salt, to taste

INSTRUCTIONS:

1. Roast chopped vegetables in the oven at 300°F until tender and set aside.

2. Cook quinoa in water until fluffy and water is absorbed (see cooking instructions on box).

3. Toss vegetables and quinoa together and serve warm or at room temperature with lemon juice and sea salt, to taste.

Chopped Salmon Salad

(1 serving)

INGREDIENTS:

6 oz can wild caught salmon, drained and flaked
1 cup romaine lettuce, chopped
1 cup raw kale, chopped
½ cup grape tomatoes, halved
½ cucumber, peeled and diced
1 tbsp sunflower seeds
extra-virgin olive oil
balsamic vinegar
sea salt and pepper, to taste

INSTRUCTIONS:

1. Combine salmon, lettuce, kale, tomatoes, cucumber and sunflower seeds in a medium bowl. Toss together.

2. Drizzle with olive oil and balsamic vinegar. Season with sea salt and pepper. Toss again.

Cool Southwest Quinoa Salad (Vegetarian)

(4 servings)

INGREDIENTS:

1 cup raw quinoa (see cooking instructions on box)
½ cup canned black beans, drained and rinsed
1 bell pepper, cored and diced
1 tbsp cilantro, minced
½ small jicama, peeled and diced
1 tsp chili powder
¼ cup apple cider vinegar

INSTRUCTIONS:

1. Cook quinoa.

2. Combine all ingredients.

3. Serve chilled.

Lentil Salad (Vegetarian)

(3–4 servings)

INGREDIENTS:

2 cups lentils, rinsed

3½ cups purified water

2–3 tbsp balsamic vinegar

½ cup extra-virgin olive oil

2 garlic cloves, minced

2 tsp dried basil

1 tsp sea salt

¼ tsp pepper

½ cup carrots, shredded

2 medium tomatoes, cut into chunks, or 1 cup cherry tomatoes

1 medium red bell pepper, cut into chunks

1 small red onion, finely chopped

1 cup fresh parsley, coarsely chopped

INSTRUCTIONS:

1. Simmer lentils in water 30–45 minutes, until cooked and cool.

2. Whisk together vinegar, olive oil, garlic, basil, sea salt and pepper.

3. Mix lentils with remaining ingredients.

4. Mix in dressing and serve.

Cool Curried Chicken Salad

(4 servings)

INGREDIENTS:

4 chicken breasts
1 cup apple, washed, unpeeled and diced
2 celery stalks, diced
½ small jicama, peeled and diced
½ cup unsweetened mango or papaya juice
1 tsp curry powder
½ tsp turmeric
1 tbsp extra-virgin olive oil
sea salt and pepper, to taste

INSTRUCTIONS:

1. Bake chicken at 350°F for 30 minutes, or until fully cooked, then dice.

2. Place chicken in a large salad bowl and cool.

3. Combine with remaining ingredients.

4. Adjust seasoning to taste and refrigerate for an hour before serving.

Salmon and Asparagus Pesto Salad

(2 servings)

INGREDIENTS:

2 salmon fillets
1 bunch asparagus, woody ends chopped off
extra-virgin olive oil
sea salt and pepper, to taste
4 cups mesclun greens or arugula
juice of 1 lemon

For the pesto:

2 bunches fresh basil, washed and leaves pulled from the hard stalks
¼ cup pine nuts
1 garlic clove
½ cup extra-virgin olive oil
sea salt, to taste

INSTRUCTIONS:

For the pesto:

1. Place the basil, pine nuts and garlic in a food processor and process on medium.

2. Slowly drizzle in olive oil while the processor is running.

3. Season with sea salt.

4. If it is too thick, add a small amount of purified water (¼ cup at most).

5. Set aside in a bowl.

(continued)

••

For the salmon and salad:

1. Turn the grill on high. (If you don't have a grill, you can use your oven's broiler or cook on your stove top on a grill pan.)

2. Brush salmon and asparagus with olive oil and season with sea salt and pepper.

3. Grill the asparagus first, for 2 minutes each side. Set aside.

4. Grill the salmon for 3 minutes on each side.

5. Prepare the salad: place the greens in a bowl, toss with olive oil, sea salt and lemon juice.

6. Place the salad on two plates and arrange the asparagus and salmon on top.

7. Drizzle 1 tbsp pesto over the top of each piece of salmon.

8. Serve while salmon is warm.

Arugula and Apricot Salad (Vegetarian)

(1 serving)

INGREDIENTS:

> 1 cup arugula
> 2–3 apricots, pitted and quartered
> 1 tbsp slivered almonds
> balsamic vinegar
> extra-virgin olive oil

INSTRUCTIONS:

1. Mix together arugula, apricots and almonds.

2. Drizzle with balsamic vinegar and olive oil.

SOUP RECIPES

Carrot and Ginger Soup (Vegetarian)

(2 servings)

INGREDIENTS:

3 cups carrots, chopped
1 medium onion, diced
½ inch ginger (plus extra for garnish), peeled and grated
6 cups purified water
sea salt, to taste
fresh parsley or dill, to finish

INSTRUCTIONS:

1. Place vegetables, ginger and water in a medium saucepan. Bring to a boil.

2. Reduce heat and allow to simmer for 15 minutes until vegetables are soft.

3. Blend ingredients to a creamy texture.

4. Add sea salt and extra ginger to taste.

5. Pour blended soup back into saucepan, reheat and serve.

6. Top with parsley or dill.

Bean Soup (Vegetarian)

(6 servings)

INGREDIENTS:

2 cups canned white kidney beans (cannellini)

1½ cups canned red kidney beans

1 cup canned garbanzo beans (chickpeas)

2–3 cups fresh spinach or escarole, washed, drained and chopped, or 10 oz frozen chopped spinach

4 cups vegetable broth

2 medium onions, chopped

1 large clove garlic, minced

3 tsp dried herbs (basil, parsley, oregano)

sea salt and pepper, to taste

INSTRUCTIONS:

1. Combine all ingredients and simmer for about 45 minutes, until onions are soft.

••

Rice and Bean Soup (Vegetarian)

(8 servings)

INGREDIENTS:

- 1 large onion, chopped
- 2 celery stalks, diced
- 3 carrots, diced
- 2 garlic cloves, minced
- 1 tbsp extra-virgin olive oil
- 6 cups vegetable stock or purified water
- 28 oz canned tomatoes with juice
- ⅓ cup brown rice
- 1 bay leaf
- 2 cups canned kidney beans
- 1 lb fresh green beans, cut into 1-inch pieces, or 10 oz frozen cut green beans

INSTRUCTIONS:

1. In a large pot, sauté onion, celery, carrots and garlic in olive oil until softened.

2. Add stock or water, tomatoes, rice and bay leaf.

3. Bring to a boil and cover.

4. Reduce heat to a simmer for 50 minutes; stir occasionally.

5. Stir in kidney beans and green beans and simmer for a further 5–10 minutes until all vegetables are tender.

6. Remove bay leaf before serving.

Escarole and White Bean Soup (Vegetarian)

(4–5 servings)

INGREDIENTS:

1 large onion, chopped
3 medium garlic cloves, crushed
1 tbsp extra-virgin olive oil
1 bay leaf
2 stalks celery, diced
1 medium carrot, diced
sea salt and pepper, to taste
5 cups vegetable broth or purified water
2 cups canned white beans
½ lb fresh escarole or spinach, chopped
freshly grated nutmeg (optional)

INSTRUCTIONS:

1. In a saucepan, sauté the onions and garlic in olive oil over medium to low heat.

2. When onions and garlic are soft, add bay leaf, celery, carrot, sea salt and pepper; stir and sauté for another 5 minutes.

3. Add broth or water and cover. Simmer for about 20 minutes.

4. Add cooked beans and escarole or spinach.

5. Cover and continue to simmer over very low heat for another 15–20 minutes.

6. If desired, season to taste with sea salt, pepper and nutmeg.

Quinoa Soup (Vegetarian)

(4–6 servings)

INGREDIENTS:

¼ cup raw quinoa, rinsed well
½ cup carrots, diced
¼ cup celery, diced
2 tbsp onion, diced
¼ cup green bell pepper, diced
2 garlic cloves, chopped
2 tsp extra-virgin olive oil
4 cups purified water
½ cup tomato, diced
½ cup cabbage, chopped
sea salt and pepper, to taste
¼ cup fresh parsley, chopped

INSTRUCTIONS:

1. Sauté quinoa, carrots, celery, onions, green bell peppers and garlic in olive oil until softened.

2. Add water, tomato and cabbage. Bring to a boil.

3. Reduce to a simmer for 20–30 minutes or until tender.

4. Season with sea salt and pepper, to taste, and garnish with parsley.

5. For variations, try adding some of your other favorite vegetables, chopped and sautéed.

Chicken and Lentil Soup

(4 servings)

INGREDIENTS:

  1 carrot, chopped
  1 onion, chopped
  1 leek, chopped
  1 celery stalk, chopped
  2 tbsp extra-virgin olive oil
  4 cups chicken broth
  1 bay leaf
  1 tbsp thyme
  ½ cup lentils
  4 chicken breasts, cooked and diced
  sea salt and pepper, to taste

INSTRUCTIONS:

1. Sauté the vegetables in the olive oil.

2. Add chicken broth and herbs and bring to a boil.

3. Simmer for 30 minutes.

4. Add lentils and simmer for a further 30 minutes.

5. Stir in the diced chicken.

6. Season with sea salt and pepper.

Spiced Butternut Squash Soup (Vegetarian)

(6 servings)

INGREDIENTS:

2 tbsp extra-virgin olive oil
1 onion, chopped
2 garlic cloves, chopped
½ tbsp turmeric
⅛ tsp cinnamon
⅛ tsp cardamom
dash of ground cloves
2 tbsp ginger, peeled and grated
2 carrots, chopped
1 tart apple, peeled, quartered and chopped
4 cups butternut squash, chopped
3 cups purified water
sea salt and pepper, to taste

INSTRUCTIONS:

1. Heat olive oil in a saucepan over medium heat.

2. Add onion and garlic cloves, cooking until tender.

3. Add the turmeric, cinnamon, cardamom, cloves and ginger, cooking until fragrant (about 1 minute).

4. Add the carrots, apple, butternut squash and water.

5. Bring to a boil, cover partially and reduce to a simmer.

6. Season with sea salt and pepper, to taste.

7. Working in batches, puree until smooth in a blender.

8. Serve warm.

••

Vegetable Soup (Vegetarian)

(6 servings)

INGREDIENTS:

2 tbsp olive oil

1 medium yellow or white onion, chopped

2 large celery stalks, chopped

3 large carrots, chopped

5 garlic cloves, minced or chopped

½ sweet potato, chopped into bite-size pieces (optional—if you omit the sweet potato, add more vegetables)

1 red bell pepper, chopped

sea salt, to taste

6 cups water or vegetable broth

¼ cup dried basil

pepper, to taste

½ cup fresh flat-leaf parsley, chopped

3 large leaves of collard greens, chopped into thin strips

*You can add your own combo of detox-friendly vegetables to change the taste and texture.

INSTRUCTIONS:

1. In a large soup pot, add olive oil and turn on stove to medium. Add onion, celery, carrots, garlic, sweet potato, red bell pepper and a pinch of sea salt. Cook until the onion has wilted and the vegetables are hot.

2. Add 6 cups of water or vegetable broth, basil, sea salt and pepper. Turn heat to high and bring to a boil. Reduce heat to medium low, cover and let simmer until vegetables are soft (about 30 minutes). Add parsley and collard greens for the last 5 minutes of cooking.

SIDE DISH RECIPES

Black Bean Salad (Vegetarian)

(4 servings)

INGREDIENTS:

2 cups canned black beans
1 cup cherry tomatoes, halved
¼ cup red onion, minced
½ cup red or yellow bell pepper, diced
1 tbsp extra-virgin olive oil
1 tsp lemon juice
1–2 tsp cumin

INSTRUCTIONS:

1. Mix all ingredients together.
2. Chill before serving.

Three Bean Salad (Vegetarian)

(4 servings)

INGREDIENTS:

½ cup canned chickpeas
½ cup canned navy beans
½ cup canned kidney beans
2 celery stalks, chopped
1 red onion, chopped
1 tbsp rosemary
1 tbsp parsley
2 tbsp extra-virgin olive oil
sea salt and pepper, to taste

INSTRUCTIONS:

1. Mix all ingredients together.

2. Chill for an hour before eating to allow the flavors to soak through.

Carrot Slaw (Vegetarian)

(4 servings)

INGREDIENTS:

2 cups carrots, shredded
½ cup celery, diced
¼ cup sunflower seeds
3–4 tbsp unsweetened coconut milk
2 tbsp unsweetened pineapple juice

INSTRUCTIONS:

1. Mix all ingredients together.
2. Chill before serving.

Red Cabbage Apple Slaw (Vegetarian)

(6 servings)

INGREDIENTS:

1 small red cabbage head, coarsely chopped
3 tart green apples, unpeeled, washed and shredded
10 radishes, shredded
2 green onions, chopped
1 celery stalk, chopped
¼ cup walnuts, chopped
1–2 tbsp lemon juice
dash garlic powder

INSTRUCTIONS:

1. Mix all ingredients together.
2. Chill for an hour before eating to allow the flavors to soak through.

••

Citrus Grilled Radicchio (Vegetarian)

(4 servings)

INGREDIENTS:

2 tbsp lemon juice
2 tbsp extra-virgin olive oil
sea salt and pepper, to taste
1 radicchio head, quartered

INSTRUCTIONS:

1. In a bowl, whisk together lemon juice, olive oil, sea salt and pepper.

2. Drizzle over the cut sides of the radicchio.

3. Grill on all sides until tender.

Oven-Roasted Vegetables (Vegetarian)

(4–6 servings)

INGREDIENTS:

1 eggplant, unpeeled and washed
1 sweet potato, unpeeled and washed
1 yellow or green summer squash
15 asparagus spears
1 red onion
3 garlic cloves, crushed
extra-virgin olive oil
3 tbsp dried herbs (rosemary, oregano, tarragon, basil, etc.)
sea salt and pepper, to taste

INSTRUCTIONS:

1. Cut all vegetables into bite-size pieces.

2. Toss vegetables with crushed garlic cloves and lightly coat vegetables with olive oil and dried herbs.

3. Spread on a roasting pan in a single layer and roast for around 20 minutes at 400°F until vegetables are tender and slightly brown, stirring occasionally.

4. Season with sea salt and pepper.

5. Serve immediately while warm.

Roasted Asparagus (Vegetarian)

(4 servings)

INGREDIENTS:

- 1 bunch asparagus
- 2 tbsp lemon zest
- ¼ cup slivered almonds
- 2 tbsp extra-virgin olive oil

INSTRUCTIONS:

1. Preheat oven to 350°F.

2. In a bowl, toss all ingredients together.

3. Lay asparagus on a sheet tray in a single layer.

4. Bake for about 20 minutes, rolling over the asparagus every 5 minutes until brown on all sides.

Rice Pilaf (Vegetarian)

(4 servings)

INGREDIENTS:

2 cups purified water
1 cup brown basmati rice
½ cup almonds
1 garlic clove
1½ tbsp extra-virgin olive oil
1½ tbsp lemon juice
½ cucumber, diced
sea salt and pepper, to taste

INSTRUCTIONS:

1. Bring water to a boil and add rice. Stir and simmer covered for 45 minutes (do not stir again).

2. Remove from heat and let sit for another 10 minutes; then remove cover and allow it to cool.

3. While rice is cooking, blend almonds, garlic, olive oil and lemon juice in a food processor.

4. When rice is cool, stir in the nut mixture and add cucumber.

5. Season with sea salt and pepper.

Sweet Potato Squash (Vegetarian)

(4–6 servings)

INGREDIENTS:

1 medium butternut squash, peeled, cut into chunks
2 medium/large sweet potatoes, peeled, cut into chunks
½ tsp ginger, grated
½ tsp cinnamon
dash nutmeg
¼ cup unsweetened coconut or almond milk

INSTRUCTIONS:

1. Preheat oven to 350°F.

2. Steam squash and sweet potato until tender; then puree in a food processor.

3. Add ginger, cinnamon, nutmeg and milk alternative (add enough to match the consistency of mashed potatoes).

4. Put mixture into casserole dish and garnish with a sprinkle of additional cinnamon.

5. Bake for about 15 minutes.

Brown Rice Risotto (Vegetarian)

(4 servings)

INGREDIENTS:

1 tbsp extra-virgin olive oil
1 medium onion, chopped
4 celery stalks, chopped
1 fennel bulb, leaves and stalks removed, chopped
½ cup brown rice
1 medium zucchini, chopped
2 cups chicken broth
1 cup purified water
sea salt, to taste

INSTRUCTIONS:

1. Add olive oil, onion, celery and fennel to a large skillet and cook until vegetables are translucent.

2. Add rice, zucchini and 1 cup of chicken broth.

3. Stir occasionally, allowing broth to be absorbed.

4. Add the second cup of broth, stirring occasionally.

5. Once absorbed, add in the water.

6. Stir and add sea salt.

7. Continue to add water if needed, until the rice reaches desired texture.

Hot Pasta Salad (Vegetarian)

(4 servings)

INGREDIENTS:

> 16 oz canned cannellini beans (reserve ½ cup liquid)
> 3 tbsp extra-virgin olive oil
> 2 onions, chopped
> 2 carrots, chopped
> 1 tsp dried oregano
> 2 tbsp dried basil
> 16 oz canned tomatoes
> 1–2 tsp sea salt
> ½ lb brown rice elbow macaroni

INSTRUCTIONS:

1. Drain beans, reserving liquid.

2. Heat 1–2 tbsp olive oil in heavy casserole dish.

3. Add onions, carrots, oregano and basil; cook until vegetables are browned.

4. Add tomatoes, bean liquid and sea salt.

5. Cover and simmer for about 10 minutes, until the vegetables are tender.

6. Add the drained beans and simmer for another 10 minutes.

7. Meanwhile, cook and drain the macaroni.

8. Toss macaroni with 1 tbsp olive oil and then mix with the bean sauce.

Nutty Green Rice (Vegetarian)

(1 serving)

INGREDIENTS:

½ cup purified water
¼ cup brown basmati rice
3 tbsp sliced almonds
parsley sprigs
1 garlic clove
½ tbsp extra-virgin olive oil
½ tsp lemon juice
½ cucumber, diced
sea salt and pepper, to taste

INSTRUCTIONS:

1. Bring water to a boil and add rice.

2. Stir and simmer covered for 45 minutes (do not stir again).

3. Remove from heat and let sit for another 10 minutes; then remove cover and allow to cool.

4. While rice is cooking, blend almonds, parsley, garlic, olive oil and lemon juice in a food processor.

5. When rice is cool, stir in the nut mixture and add cucumber. Add sea salt and pepper, to taste.

Healthy Raw Ketchup

(about 2½ cups)

INGREDIENTS:

- 1 cup tomato, chopped
- 1 cup sun-dried tomatoes, soaked for 30 minutes, drained and chopped
- 1 tbsp garlic, minced
- 10 fresh basil leaves
- 3 dates, pitted
- 1–2 tbsp Bragg's raw, unfiltered apple cider vinegar
- ¼ cup extra-virgin olive oil
- 1 tsp sea salt

INSTRUCTIONS:

1. Blend all ingredients together until it forms a paste.

DESSERTS

Baked Apples (Vegetarian)

(2 servings)

INGREDIENTS:

2 apples
½ cup unsweetened apple juice
½ tsp cinnamon

INSTRUCTIONS:

1. Core apples and peel only the top ⅓ of the skin.
2. Place in baking dish; pour apple juice over the apples and sprinkle with cinnamon.
3. Bake at 350°F for 20–30 minutes, until soft and juicy.

Grilled Strawberries (Vegetarian)

(1 serving)

INGREDIENTS:

½ cup strawberries, halved
walnut oil
balsamic vinegar (optional)

INSTRUCTIONS:

1. Brush strawberries with walnut oil and grill.
2. Try drizzling with a little bit of balsamic vinegar.

Grilled Figs (Vegetarian)

(1 serving)

INGREDIENTS:

　　3 figs, halved
　　walnut oil
　　balsamic vinegar (optional)

INSTRUCTIONS:

1. Brush figs with walnut oil and grill.

2. Try drizzling with a little bit of balsamic vinegar.

Nb & B Snack (Vegetarian)

(1 serving)

INGREDIENTS:

　　2 tbsp nut butter
　　⅓ cup berries, sliced if necessary
　　1 brown rice cake

INSTRUCTIONS:

1. Layer ingredients on rice cake in order listed.

SAVORY SNACKS

Kale Chips (Vegetarian)

(2 servings)

INGREDIENTS:

1 bunch of kale, washed and dried well
2 tsp of extra-virgin olive oil
sea salt, to taste

INSTRUCTIONS:

1. Preheat oven to 350°F.

2. Remove the stem for each kale leaf and rip or cut the leaves into bite-size pieces. There's no need to be precise or exact; you can make them however big or small you like.

3. Place kale in a large bowl and toss with olive oil and sea salt.

4. Massage the olive oil into the kale, making sure each piece is lightly coated.

5. Spread kale out amongst two rimmed baking sheets, being sure not to overlap any of the pieces. It is important that your kale is in a single layer because if the leaves are piled on top of each other they will steam rather than bake which means they won't get crunchy.

6. Bake for about 15 minutes, until the leaves are crispy and crunchy.

Roasted Chickpeas (Vegetarian)

(4 servings)

INGREDIENTS:

12 oz canned chickpeas (garbanzo beans), drained
2 tbsp extra-virgin olive oil
sea salt, to taste
cayenne pepper (optional)

INSTRUCTIONS:

1. Preheat oven to 450°F.

2. Blot chickpeas with a paper towel to dry them.

3. In a bowl, toss chickpeas with olive oil and season to taste with sea salt and cayenne pepper.

4. Spread on a baking sheet and bake for 30–40 minutes, until browned and crunchy. Watch carefully for the last few minutes to avoid burning.

Caprese Snack (Vegetarian)

(1 serving)

INGREDIENTS:

- 1–2 tbsp walnut "cheese" (soak walnuts in purified water for 2 hours and puree; can be stored in fridge)
- 1–2 basil leaves
- 1 large or 2 small tomato slices
- sea salt and pepper, to taste
- 1 brown rice cake

INSTRUCTIONS:

1. Layer ingredients on rice cake in order listed.

Guacamole (Vegetarian)

(6 servings)

INGREDIENTS:

- 3 avocados
- juice of ½ lime
- ½ red onion, minced
- 1 tbsp cilantro, chopped
- 1 garlic clove, minced
- sea salt and pepper, to taste
- *Can also add chopped tomato and/or chopped jalapeño pepper for extra flavor

INSTRUCTIONS:

1. Take the flesh from the avocados and mix in a bowl with the rest of the ingredients.
2. Mush all ingredients together to desired texture.

Classic Hummus (Vegetarian)

(6 servings)

INGREDIENTS:

2 cups canned garbanzo beans (chickpeas)
¼ cup tahini (optional)
1 tsp cumin
⅓ cup lemon juice
2 tbsp extra-virgin olive oil or flaxseed oil
2 garlic cloves, crushed
sea salt, to taste

INSTRUCTIONS:

1. Drain beans and reserve liquid.

2. Blend beans in a food processor with remaining ingredients.

3. If mixture seems dry, add some of the reserved liquid slowly to the blender to make a smooth paste.

Garlic Hummus (Vegetarian)

Same as above, but replace olive oil in recipe with garlic oil.

Roasted Garlic Oil (Vegetarian)

INGREDIENTS:

extra-virgin olive oil
garlic

INSTRUCTIONS:

1. Place olive oil and garlic cloves in an oven-safe container like a bread pan and bake at 350°F until garlic is soft.

2. Store in a sealed jar, leaving in the cloves to soak.

SHAKES & SMOOTHIES

These recipes for shakes and smoothies should be made with your favorite protein powder. For best results, mix in this order:

1) add liquids

2) add powders

3) add fruit

Preferred milk alternatives are almond, coconut and hemp milk. Rice milk can be used, but it has a greater impact on blood sugar.

Shake Recipes (No Fruit)

Coconut

4 oz unsweetened coconut milk
4 oz water or 4 oz water and ½ cup ice

Almond Crunch

4 oz unsweetened almond milk and ½ cup ice
1–2 tbsp sliced or slivered raw almonds
1 tsp xylitol or agave nectar (if needed)

Almond

4 oz unsweetened almond milk
4 oz water or 4 oz water and ½ cup ice

Horchata

Vanilla PhysioMeal
4 oz water or unsweetened rice milk
½ cup ice
1 tsp cinnamon

Cherry Spice

Use Strawberry PhysioMeal
4 oz water or unsweetened milk alternative
4 oz unsweetened organic cherry juice
½ cup ice
2 tsp grated ginger
1 tsp cinnamon

Smoothie Recipes

Basic Berry

4 oz water or unsweetened milk alternative
½ cup frozen organic berries

Coco-Nutty

4 oz unsweetened coconut milk and ½ cup ice
3 tbsp shredded organic coconut
1 tsp xylitol or agave nectar (if needed)

Black and Cran

4 oz unsweetened milk alternative
½ cup ice
¼–½ cup unsweetened organic cranberries and blackberries

• •

Lemon-Lime

4 oz unsweetened milk alternative and ½ cup ice
½ lemon/lime (peeled and sliced)
*may add a few lemon and lime rind shavings for health and taste,
    or use 1–2 tbsp lemon-lime juice to taste

Apricot-Raspberry

4 oz unsweetened milk alternative
½ cup fresh or water-packed organic apricots
½ cup frozen organic raspberries
pinch of cinnamon

Piña Colada

4 oz coconut water
4 oz water or ½ cup ice
½–1 cup frozen organic pineapple or mango
1–2 tsp shredded organic coconut

Berry Berry

4 oz unsweetened milk alternative
4 oz water or ½ cup ice
½–1 cup frozen organic raspberries, strawberries and/or
    blueberries

Coconut Freeze (Requires Planning)

4 oz unsweetened coconut milk
½ organic banana, frozen

South Side

4 oz unsweetened milk alternative
½ cup frozen organic peaches
1 tbsp flaxseed, ground
2 tsp freshly grated ginger
pinch of cinnamon

Moderate Carbohydrate Content Smoothies

The following smoothies are delicious but have slightly more carbs than the ones listed above.

Peaches-n-Cream

4 oz unsweetened milk alternative
4 oz water or ½ cup ice
½ cup organic fresh peaches

Apple-Pecan Spice

4 oz unsweetened milk alternative
4 oz water or ½ cup ice
½ cup unsweetened organic apple sauce
¼ cup raw pecans, slivered (can substitute sliced raw almonds)
cinnamon, to taste

Apple Spice

4 oz unsweetened milk alternative
4 oz water or ½ cup ice
½ cup unsweetened organic apple sauce
cinnamon, to taste

Green Smoothie

Greens Mojito

INGREDIENTS:

2 slices organic cucumber
2 sprigs fresh mint
4 oz coconut water

4 oz water
1 scoop PhysioGreens
slice of lemon

INSTRUCTIONS:

1. Muddle the cucumber and fresh mint together, add coconut water, water and PhysioGreens and mix well. Garnish with lemon.

The Smart Way to Snack

IF NEEDED, YOU MAY HAVE UP TO TWO SNACKS PER DAY.

It is important to *only* snack when you are hungry. In general people tend to snack when they are stressed, tired, thirsty or bored. Make yourself wait fifteen minutes before eating.

Snacks should be about half the size of a regular meal.

Remember to eat a protein with every snack (chicken, turkey, hard-boiled egg, nuts, nut butters, etc.).

Smoothies: If you have a smoothie instead of a shake, try to snack mainly on protein sources (nuts, fish, chicken, eggs, etc.) and limit the amount of carbohydrates since the fruit included in the smoothie already counts as carbohydrates.

Shakes: If you have a shake (no fruits), you can have carbohydrates (fruits and nongluten grains) with your protein sources.

Snack Suggestions

- Mixed raw nuts and seeds with unsweetened, unsulfured dried fruit
- Wild caught canned tuna or salmon mixed with hummus with rice crackers
- Grilled chicken breast with hummus
- Hard-boiled egg; celery dipped in hummus
- Deviled eggs—remove yolk and replace with hummus and sprinkle with paprika
- Apple with almond butter or handful of raw nuts
- Berries and raw nuts
- Raw nuts and/or seeds

- ½ MacroBar, ½ PranaBar or other clean detox bar (avoid the ones with chocolate or peanuts)
- Sliced turkey (from Whole Foods fresh deli or similar—make sure it is 100 percent plain turkey breast, no maple syrup, etc.) with hummus on a rice cake
- Grilled chicken with quinoa
- Celery sticks with nut butter
- Grilled chicken with sliced avocado; sprinkle with sea salt
- Gluten- and yeast-free bread with almond butter and cinnamon

25AL ROKER

MY PERSONAL FAVORITES!

The following recipes are some of my favorite classics I prepare for family and friends. They are healthy, delicious and a pleasant break from eating perfectly all the time—although they're still healthy and delicious! I hope you enjoy them as much as I do!

Guacamole

(8 servings or 3 cups)

Tip: Don't try to make this more than 2 hours in advance; it will turn a very unappealing shade of brown.

INGREDIENTS:

3 ripe avocados
3 tbsp freshly squeezed lime juice (from 1–2 limes)
½ large tomato, stemmed
½ large onion, peeled and finely chopped
2 cloves garlic, peeled and minced
½ jalapeño pepper, stemmed, seeded and finely chopped
½ cup chopped cilantro leaves
1 tsp coarse salt, such as kosher salt
fresh cracked pepper

INSTRUCTIONS:

1. Using a sharp knife, cut the avocados in half. Remove the pits. Scoop the flesh into a medium bowl and roughly crush with a potato masher or fork. Stir in the lime juice.

2. Chop the tomato as finely as possible. Scrape the tomato flesh and juice into the bowl with the avocados.

3. Add the onion, garlic, jalapeño pepper, cilantro, salt and pepper, and stir to mix.

4. Press a sheet of plastic wrap on the surface of the guacamole. Let sit for about 30 minutes at room temperature and then adjust the seasonings; you may want to add more jalapeño pepper, lime juice, salt or pepper.

5. Serve at room temperature with tortilla chips for dipping.

Black Bean Dip

(8 servings or 3 cups)

INGREDIENTS:

2 (15½ oz) cans black beans, drained, rinsed and drained again
1 cup cilantro leaves, chopped
2 tbsp orange zest (from 2 oranges), finely grated
⅓ cup freshly squeezed orange juice (from 1 orange)
¼ cup canola oil or other vegetable oil
1 tsp salt
several dashes Louisiana-style hot sauce

INSTRUCTIONS:

1. Put all of the ingredients in the work bowl of a food processor or in a blender (you may have to do this in 2 batches if using a blender), and puree until smooth. Transfer to a bowl and let sit for at least 30 minutes for the flavors to blend. Taste and add more salt or hot sauce, if desired.

2. This is best served the day you make it, but you can keep the dip for up to 2 days in a covered container in the refrigerator. Serve at room temperature with wedges of pita bread.

••

Spinach-Yogurt Dip

(8 servings or 3 cups)

INGREDIENTS:

1 (10 oz) package frozen chopped spinach, thawed
½ small onion, peeled and halved
2 cloves garlic, peeled
1 cup plain yogurt
1 cup low-fat sour cream
½ tsp salt
freshly ground pepper

INSTRUCTIONS:

1. Put the spinach in a colander and, using your hands or the back of a spoon, squeeze out as much liquid as possible. Set the spinach aside.

2. If using a food processor, put the onion and garlic in the bowl and pulse until finely chopped. Add the yogurt, sour cream, salt, pepper and the spinach, and puree until smooth. If using a blender, chop the onion and garlic roughly by hand, then put in the blender along with the remaining ingredients. Process until smooth.

3. Cover and refrigerate for at least 1 hour or up to 24 hours before serving. Serve with sliced raw vegetables and wedges of pita bread.

Vegetarian Burgers

(4 servings)

INGREDIENTS:

4 large portobello mushrooms
2 tbsp extra-virgin olive oil
salt
freshly ground pepper
2 large red bell peppers (see note)
8 large slices crusty bread, preferably sourdough
4 oz herbed cheese spread or fresh goat cheese
12 large spinach leaves, stemmed, rinsed and dried

INSTRUCTIONS:

1. Prepare a charcoal fire or preheat a gas grill for direct grilling so that you have a medium-heat and a high-heat area.

2. While the grill is heating, stem the mushrooms. You can leave the dark gills on the underside; they give the mushrooms a more intense flavor. If you choose to remove the gills, use the edge of a teaspoon to scoop them out. Wipe the mushrooms clean with a damp paper towel. Using a pastry brush, generously coat both sides of each mushroom with olive oil, and season with salt and pepper. Set the mushrooms aside.

3. Put the whole peppers on the high-heat area of the grill, and roast, turning frequently until the skin over all of the peppers turns black, about 20 minutes. Using tongs, remove the peppers from the grill, and place them in a heavy-duty, resealable plastic bag. Close the bag, and allow the peppers to cool somewhat.

4. When they're cool enough to handle, remove the charred skin from the peppers and discard. Stem and seed the peppers, and cut each into 4 pieces.

5. Grill the mushrooms over medium heat for about 15 minutes, turning once, until they are well browned and softened.

••

6. While the mushrooms are grilling, toast the bread lightly over the high-heat area of the grill, about 1 minute per side. Remove the bread from the grill and spread about 1 tsp of the cheese over each slice.

7. Using tongs, remove a mushroom from the grill and place it on a piece of bread spread with cheese. Top with 2 pieces of the red pepper and 3 spinach leaves; then place a second piece of bread, cheese side down, on top. Repeat with the remaining ingredients, until you have made 4 sandwiches.

Note: You may substitute 1 (8 oz) jar of roasted red peppers, drained, for the fresh peppers, and skip the roasting step.

Grilled Chicken Breasts, Any Way, Any Day

(6 servings)

INGREDIENTS:

6 (6-oz) boneless, skinless chicken breast halves
White Wine–Tarragon Marinade or Honey-Mustard Marinade
   (see p. 266)

INSTRUCTIONS:

1. Rinse the chicken under cold running water and pat dry with paper towels. Put the chicken pieces in a shallow, nonreactive pan and pour the marinade over the chicken. Turn each piece to coat. Cover and refrigerate for at least 4 hours, or up to 12 hours, turning once during this time. Let sit at room temperature for 20 minutes before grilling.

2. Prepare a charcoal fire or preheat a gas grill for direct grilling over medium heat.

3. Remove the chicken from the pan and discard the marinade. Grill the chicken for 6–8 minutes per side, until the outside is well browned, the meat is no longer pink when pierced and an instant-read thermometer inserted into the center reads 170°F. Serve immediately.

White Wine–Tarragon Marinade

(1½ cups or enough for up to 4 lbs of chicken or seafood)

INGREDIENTS:

¾ cup white wine or white vermouth

6 tbsp extra-virgin olive oil

6 tbsp freshly squeezed lemon juice (from 2 lemons)

6 cloves garlic, peeled and chopped

2 tbsp chopped tarragon leaves or 1 tbsp dried tarragon

1½ tsp coarse salt, such as kosher salt

1 tsp freshly ground pepper

INSTRUCTIONS:

1. In a small bowl, whisk together all of the ingredients. Use immediately, or cover and store in the refrigerator for up to 2 days.

Honey-Mustard Marinade

(about 1 cup or enough for up to 3 lbs of chicken or pork)

INGREDIENTS:

½ cup honey

¼ cup Dijon mustard

¼ cup freshly squeezed lemon juice (from 1–2 lemons)

4 tsp soy sauce

3 garlic cloves, peeled and chopped

INSTRUCTIONS:

1. In a small bowl, whisk together all of the ingredients. Use immediately, or cover and store in the refrigerator for up to 2 days.

• •

Kebabs Cooked Right

(6 servings)

INGREDIENTS:

For the meat:

2 lbs of lamb, beef, pork, or chicken, cut into 2-inch chunks
marinade of your choice

For the vegetables:

2 lbs of assorted vegetables such as bell peppers (all colors),
   mushrooms, leeks, onions, zucchini and summer squash, cut in
   1½-inch pieces; and cherry tomatoes
⅓ cup extra-virgin olive oil
2 tbsp freshly squeezed lemon juice (from 1 lemon)
salt
freshly ground pepper

INSTRUCTIONS:

1. Place the meat in a shallow, nonreactive pan and pour the marinade over it. Cover the pan and refrigerate for at least 8 hours and up to 24 hours, turning once during this time.

2. Prepare a charcoal fire or preheat a gas grill for direct grilling, so that you can have a medium-heat and a high-heat area. If using bamboo skewers, soak them in water for at least 15 minutes to prevent them from burning.

3. Remove the meat from the pan, discard the marinade and thread the meat onto skewers. Make sure to leave a bit of space between the pieces, so that each piece cooks through.

4. In a bowl, toss the vegetables with the oil, lemon juice, salt and pepper. Thread them onto skewers. You can mix them up, except for the tomatoes, which should be skewered separately.

5. Grill the meat over high heat for 12–15 minutes, turning the kebabs as they cook. Remove a chunk of meat from a skewer and slice it in half to see if it is cooked; beef and lamb can be pink inside, pork can be slightly pink, and chicken should be white throughout.

6. While the meat is cooking, grill the vegetables over medium heat, turning, for 8–10 minutes (4 minutes for cherry tomatoes). Serve immediately.

Fish Fillets with Lemon-Parsley Sauce

(4 servings)

INGREDIENTS:

For the sauce:

½ cup parsley leaves, chopped
⅓ cup extra-virgin olive oil
1½ tsp lemon zest (from 1 lemon), finely grated
3 tbsp freshly squeezed lemon juice (from 1 lemon)
2 tbsp capers, drained
salt, to taste
freshly ground pepper, to taste

For the fish:

2 lbs fish fillets such as cod, catfish, haddock, halibut, hake or
monkfish
2 to 3 tbsp extra-virgin olive oil
salt, to taste
freshly ground pepper, to taste

INSTRUCTIONS:

For the sauce:

1. Whisk together all of the ingredients in a small bowl. Cover and refrigerate until ready to use, at least 1 hour, and up to 8 hours, to let the flavors blend.

For the fish:

1. Prepare a charcoal fire or preheat a gas grill for direct grilling over high heat. If you do not have a grill basket, lay a piece of oiled, heavy-duty aluminum foil—slightly larger than the fish—on the grill, and poke several holes in it.

• •

2. Using a pastry brush, generously coat both sides of the fish with oil; then season with salt and pepper.

3. Place the fish on the grill, either in the grill basket or on the foil. If the fish has skin, place it skin side down. If using a grill basket, turn the fish once during grilling; if using the foil, do not turn it. Grill until the fish flakes when poked with a fork but is still a bit opaque in the center. The grilling time will vary according to the thickness of the fillets, but it should not take longer than 12 minutes total.

4. Transfer the fish to a platter and drizzle with some of the lemon-parsley sauce. Serve with traditional sauce on the side. The fish is excellent with grilled asparagus.

New Orleans–Style Barbecued Shrimp

(8 main-course servings or 12 appetizer servings)

INGREDIENTS:

- 4 lbs fresh or frozen large or extra-large shrimp (21–25 count per lb), in the shell
- 5 tbsp chili powder
- 1 tbsp plus 2 tsp salt
- 16 tbsp (2 sticks) unsalted butter
- 2 medium onions, peeled and freshly chopped
- 6 garlic cloves, peeled and minced
- 1 cup ketchup
- ½ cup extra-virgin olive oil
- 5 tbsp light brown sugar
- ¼ cup Worcestershire sauce
- 1 lemon, sliced
- 3 tbsp freshly squeezed lemon juice (from 1 lemon)
- 3 bay leaves
- 2 tsp dried oregano
- 2 tsp dried thyme
- 1 tsp cayenne pepper
- several dashes Louisiana-style hot sauce

INSTRUCTIONS:

1. You can buy large frozen tiger shrimp that have been deveined but are still in the shell. If you use these, thaw them according to the package directions. If using fresh shrimp, you can ask the person at the fish counter to devein them for you in the shell. You can also do this yourself, using kitchen shears: Cut the shell along the vein and pull the vein out with your fingers. Or you can just skip the deveining process. The vein won't hurt you.

2. Combine 3 tbsp of the chili powder and 1 tbsp of the salt in a small bowl. Rub the shrimp with this mixture, making sure you

rub some into the open cut where the shrimp has been deveined (if it has) to season the shrimp inside the shell. Place the shrimp in a shallow, nonreactive pan, cover with plastic wrap, and refrigerate while you make the sauce.

3. In a saucepan set over medium-high heat, melt the butter. Add the onion and garlic and cook for 3–5 minutes, until soft but not browned. Add the ketchup, oil, brown sugar, Worcestershire sauce, lemon slices, lemon juice, bay leaves, oregano, thyme, cayenne pepper and hot sauce, as well as the remaining 2 tbsp chili powder and 2 tsp salt. Stir to mix. Reduce the heat to a simmer, and cook, covered, stirring occasionally, for about 20 minutes, or until thick. Remove from the heat, uncover and cool to room temperature. Remove and discard the lemon slices and bay leaves.

4. Pour 1½ cups of the sauce over the shrimp. Toss to coat well. Cover and refrigerate the remaining sauce separately and save for dipping.

5. Prepare a charcoal fire or preheat a gas grill for direct grilling over high heat.

6. While the grill is heating, reheat the remaining sauce in a small, covered saucepan over very low heat—it will only take a few minutes. Watch the sauce carefully so that it doesn't burn.

7. Remove the shrimp from the pan and discard the marinade. Grill the shrimp for 2–3 minutes per side, until the shells are orange-pink. To test for doneness, take a shrimp off the grill, remove the shell, and cut the shrimp in half. The flesh should be white and firm throughout.

8. Serve with the warm sauce for dipping, and a large bowl for the shells.

My Mom's Peas and Rice

(8 servings)

INGREDIENTS:

½ lb salt pork, cut into 4 chunks

1 medium onion, peeled and finely chopped

6 garlic cloves, peeled and minced

1 green bell pepper, stemmed, seeded and finely chopped

3 cups white rice

6 cups water

salt, to taste

freshly ground pepper, to taste

3 (15 oz) cans red kidney beans, drained, rinsed and drained again

INSTRUCTIONS:

1. Place a large pot over medium-high heat, and add the salt pork. Cook for several minutes, until the pork renders a tbsp or so of fat. Add the onion, garlic, and bell pepper to the pot, lower the heat to medium low and continue to cook, stirring, until the onions are translucent, 5–7 minutes.

2. Add the rice to the pot and stir to combine. Pour in the water and season with salt and pepper. Bring to a boil over high heat; then reduce the heat to a simmer and cook, covered, for 20 minutes.

3. Stir the beans into the rice and cook for 10 minutes more. Remove the salt pork and discard. Serve immediately.

Corn, Black Bean and Tomato Salad

(6 servings)

INGREDIENTS:

For the dressing:

3 tbsp freshly squeezed lime juice (from 1–2 limes)
3 tbsp rice vinegar
3 tbsp peanut oil
½ tsp sugar
¼ tsp hot red pepper flakes
salt, to taste

For the salad:

2 ears corn, husked
1 (19 oz) can black beans, drained, rinsed and drained again
2 medium tomatoes (¾ pound), cored and chopped
1 large shallot, peeled and finely chopped
¼ cup cilantro leaves, chopped

INSTRUCTIONS:

For the dressing:

1. In a small bowl, whisk together all of the ingredients. Cover and refrigerate until needed or for up to 2 days.

For the salad:

1. Prepare a charcoal fire or preheat a gas grill for direct cooking over high heat.

2. Grill the corn for 8–12 minutes, until the kernels look toasty and a few are dark brown. When cool enough to handle, cut a small slice off the fattest end of the corn. Stand the ear on the flat end

in a medium bowl and, using a sharp knife, cut the corn off the cob. You should have about 2 cups of kernels.

3. Add the black beans, tomatoes, shallot and cilantro to the bowl, and mix gently. Drizzle with the dressing, and mix again. Let sit at room temperature for at least 30 minutes or up to 2 hours for the flavors to blend before serving.

A Note on My Cleanse

There are a number of cleanses on the market—some good ones and some not so good. In an effort to help you decide if a cleanse is right for you, I highly recommend checking out the Physio-Cleanse and Detoxification Program, which is the exact cleanse that Melissa Bowman Li created for her clients and the one that I personally follow at least twice a year. I have found this cleanse to be the most doable. It never felt too extreme to me, because you get to eat food and balance your nutrition through smoothies and supplements.

Although the prospect of starting a cleanse can be scary, try to stick with it, and remember, it takes at least a week to get into the rhythm. Once you do that, it becomes much easier.

For more information about the PhysioCleanse, visit the Web site at www.physiolifestudios.com. Tell Melissa that Al sent you!

About the Author

Al Roker is known to more than thirty million TV viewers, and he is the recipient of thirteen Emmy Awards, ten of which he won for his work on NBC's *Today*. He is the *New York Times* bestselling author of *Don't Make Me Stop This Car!: Adventures in Fatherhood*. An accomplished cook, Roker also has two bestselling cookbooks to his credit. Al Roker lives in Manhattan with his wife, ABC News and *20/20* correspondent Deborah Roberts, and has two daughters and a son.

CONNECT ONLINE
www.alroker.com
twitter.com/#alroker